T0348727

# Top 10 Primary Care Training Room Conditions

*Editors*

SIOBHAN M. STATUTA
JOHN M. MACKNIGHT

# CLINICS IN
# SPORTS MEDICINE

www.sportsmed.theclinics.com

*Consulting Editor*
MARK D. MILLER

October 2019 • Volume 38 • Number 4

**ELSEVIER**

1600 John F. Kennedy Boulevard • Suite 1800 • Philadelphia, Pennsylvania, 19103-2899

http://www.theclinics.com

**CLINICS IN SPORTS MEDICINE Volume 38, Number 4**
**October 2019 ISSN 0278-5919, ISBN-13: 978-0-323-67222-1**

Editor: Lauren Boyle
Developmental Editor: Donald Mumford

© **2019 Elsevier Inc. All rights reserved.**

This periodical and the individual contributions contained in it are protected under copyright by Elsevier, and the following terms and conditions apply to their use:

**Photocopying**

Single photocopies of single articles may be made for personal use as allowed by national copyright laws. Permission of the Publisher and payment of a fee is required for all other photocopying, including multiple or systematic copying, copying for advertising or promotional purposes, resale, and all forms of document delivery. Special rates are available for educational institutions that wish to make photocopies for non-profit educational classroom use. For information on how to seek permission visit www.elsevier.com/permissions or call: (+44) 1865 843830 (UK)/(+1) 215 239 3804 (USA).

**Derivative Works**

Subscribers may reproduce tables of contents or prepare lists of articles including abstracts for internal circulation within their institutions. Permission of the Publisher is required for resale or distribution outside the institution. Permission of the Publisher is required for all other derivative works, including compilations and translations (please consult www.elsevier.com/permissions).

**Electronic Storage or Usage**

Permission of the Publisher is required to store or use electronically any material contained in this periodical, including any article or part of an article (please consult www.elsevier.com/permissions). Except as outlined above, no part of this publication may be reproduced, stored in a retrieval system or transmitted in any form or by any means, electronic, mechanical, photocopying, recording or otherwise, without prior written permission of the Publisher.

**Notice**

No responsibility is assumed by the Publisher for any injury and/or damage to persons or property as a matter of products liability, negligence or otherwise, or from any use or operation of any methods, products, instructions or ideas contained in the material herein. Because of rapid advances in the medical sciences, in particular, independent verification of diagnoses and drug dosages should be made.

Although all advertising material is expected to conform to ethical (medical) standards, inclusion in this publication does not constitute a guarantee or endorsement of the quality or value of such product or of the claims made of it by its manufacturer.

*Clinics in Sports Medicine* (ISSN 0278-5919) is published quarterly by Elsevier Inc., 360 Park Avenue South, New York, NY 10010-1710. Months of issue are January, April, July, and October. Business and Editorial Offices: 1600 John F. Kennedy Blvd., Ste. 1800, Philadelphia, PA 19103-2899. Customer Service Office: 3251 Riverport Lane, Maryland Heights, MO 63043. Periodicals postage paid at New York, NY and additional mailing offices. Subscription prices are $364.00 per year (US individuals), $698.00 per year (US institutions), $100.00 per year (US students), $405.00 per year (Canadian individuals), $861.00 per year (Canadian institutions), $235.00 (Canadian students), $475.00 per year (foreign individuals), $861.00 per year (foreign institutions), and $235.00 per year (foreign students). Foreign air speed delivery is included in all *Clinics* subscription prices. All prices are subject to change without notice. **POSTMASTER:** Send address changes to *Clinics in Sports Medicine*, Elsevier Health Sciences Division, Subscription Customer Service, 3251 Riverport Lane, Maryland Heights, MO 63043. Customer Service (orders, claims, online, change of address): Elsevier Health Sciences Division, Subscription Customer Service, 3251 Riverport Lane, Maryland Heights, MO 63043. **Tel: 1-800-654-2452 (U.S. and Canada); 314-447-8871 (outside U.S. and Canada). Fax: 314-447-8029. E-mail: journalscustomerservice-usa@elsevier.com (for print support); journalsonlinesupport-usa@elsevier.com (for online support).**

*Reprints.* For copies of 100 or more of articles in this publication, please contact the Commercial Reprints Department, Elsevier Inc., 360 Park Avenue South, New York, NY 10010-1710. Tel.: 212-633-3874; Fax: 212-633-3820; E-mail: reprints@elsevier.com.

*Clinics in Sports Medicine* is covered in *MEDLINE/PubMed (Index Medicus) Current Contents/Clinical Medicine, Excerpta Medica,* and *ISI/Biomed.*

# Contributors

## CONSULTING EDITOR

**MARK D. MILLER, MD**
S. Ward Casscells Professor, Head, Department of Orthopaedic Surgery, Division of Sports Medicine, University of Virginia, Charlottesville, Virginia; Team Physician, Miller Review Course, Harrisonburg, Virginia

## EDITORS

**SIOBHAN M. STATUTA, MD**
Director, Primary Care Sports Medicine Fellowship, Associate Professor, Departments of Family Medicine and Physical Medicine and Rehabilitation, Team Physician, University of Virginia Sports Medicine, University of Virginia Health System, Charlottesville, Virginia

**JOHN M. MacKNIGHT, MD, FACSM**
Professor, Internal Medicine and Orthopaedic Surgery, Team Physician and Medical Director, University of Virginia Sports Medicine, University of Virginia Health System, Charlottesville, Virginia

## AUTHORS

**KELLEY ANDERSON, DO**
Department of Orthopaedic Surgery, University of Pittsburgh Medical Center, Assistant Professor of Sports Medicine, University of Pittsburgh, Pittsburgh, Pennsylvania

**ROBERT BATTLE, MD**
Division of Cardiology, University of Virginia, Charlottesville, Virginia

**JEFFREY R. BYTOMSKI, DO**
Departments of Community and Family and Medicine, and Orthopedics, Duke University, Durham, North Carolina

**PATRICK C. CARR, MD**
Department of Dermatology, University of Virginia, Charlottesville, Virginia

**ANTHONY S. CERAULO, DO**
Departments of Community and Family and Medicine, and Orthopedics, Duke University, Durham, North Carolina

**MARIO CIOCCA, MD**
Assistant Professor, Orthopeadics and Internal Medicine, Director, UNC Sports Medicine, The University of North Carolina at Chapel Hill, Chapel Hill, North Carolina

**MICHAEL COLLINS, PhD**
Professor, Department of Orthopaedic Surgery, University of Pittsburgh Medical Center
Sports Medicine Concussion Program, University of Pittsburgh Medical Center,
Pittsburgh, Pennsylvania

**THOMAS G. CROPLEY, MD**
Professor, Department of Dermatology, University of Virginia, Charlottesville,
Virginia

**PETER N. DEAN, MD**
Division of Pediatric Cardiology, Department of Pediatrics, University of Virginia,
Charlottesville, Virginia

**JEANNE DOPERAK, DO**
Department of Orthopaedic Surgery, University of Pittsburgh Medical Center, Assistant
Professor of Sports Medicine, University of Pittsburgh, Pittsburgh, Pennsylvania

**KAREN P. EGAN, PhD**
Associate Sport Psychologist, University of Virginia Athletics Department, McCue Center,
Charlottesville, Virginia

**KOUROS EMAMI, PsyD**
Neuropsychology Fellow, University of Pittsburgh Medical Center Sports Medicine
Concussion Program, Pittsburgh, Pennsylvania

**DAVID R. ESPINOZA, MD**
Department of Orthopaedics, University of Pittsburgh, Pittsburgh, Pennsylvania

**ROBERT WARNE FITCH, MD**
Associate Professor of Orthopedics and Rehab, Associate Professor of Emergency
Medicine, Vanderbilt Head Team Physician, Nashville, Tennessee

**ARMANDO GONZALEZ, MD**
Department of Orthopaedics, University of Pittsburgh, Pittsburgh, Pennsylvania

**CARRIE A. JAWORSKI, MD, FAAFP, FACSM**
Director of Primary Care Sports Medicine Fellowship, University of Chicago/NorthShore
University HealthSystem, Division Head, Primary Care Sports Medicine,
NorthShore University HealthSystem, Glenview, Illinois; Clinical Assistant
Professor of Family Medicine, University of Chicago Pritzker School of Medicine,
Chicago, Illinois

**JONATHAN H. KIM, MD, MSc**
Division of Cardiology, Emory Clinical Cardiovascular Research Institute, Emory
University School of Medicine, Atlanta, Georgia

**AARON V. MARES, MD**
Department of Orthopaedics, University of Pittsburgh, Pittsburgh, Pennsylvania

**KELLI PUGH, MS, ATC, LMT**
Associate Athletics Director for Sports Medicine, University of Virginia, Charlottesville,
Virginia

**VALERIE RYGIEL, DO**
Sports Medicine Fellow, University of Chicago/NorthShore University HealthSystem
Primary Care Sports Medicine Fellowship, Glenview, Illinois

**SIOBHAN M. STATUTA, MD**
Director, Primary Care Sports Medicine Fellowship, Associate Professor, Departments of Family Medicine and Physical Medicine and Rehabilitation, Team Physician, University of Virginia Sports Medicine, University of Virginia Health System, Charlottesville, Virginia

**JASON WILLIAMS, MD**
Vanderbilt Orthopedics Sports Medicine Fellow, Nashville, Tennessee

Downloaded

# Contents

Cardiac disease can present in the training room through three portals: the preparticipation history and physical may identify concerns, the athlete may present with symptoms, or screening modalities may demonstrate abnormal findings. Training-related cardiovascular remodeling can mimic real disease, therefore providers must be able to separate the two. Sports medicine providers must be knowledgeable in how these present and how to care for these concerns to ensure proper care and avoid unnecessary restrictions of athletes. This article discusses 10 common cardiac concerns that can arise in the training room.

Concussion is a challenging and controversial medical diagnosis that can test even the most seasoned practitioner. Knowledge on this topic is ever evolving. It was not so long ago that grading guidelines were based on loss of consciousness and amnesia. Medicine has seen a renaissance of discovery over the past 20 years in concussion evaluation and management. A PubMed search for "concussion" between 1990 and 2000 produced just over 1000 articles and that same search including the last 18 years expands to over 10,000 publications. The most recent knowledge and recommendations are discussed based on the published evidence.

The athletic training room is filled with a multitude of conditions encompassing many different specialties of medicine. When it comes to traumatic injuries in the training room, many of them are not musculoskeletal in nature. Ultrasound in the training room can help identify serious and subtle solid-organ injury and small pneumothoraces. The discussion of these conditions follows a simple outline that helps identify injury/conditions through a proper history and physical. Evidence-based treatment/management/return to play guidelines are discussed.

Although athletics participation provides benefits that can be protective for mental health, stressors unique to athletics are present. This article reviews the frequency and symptoms of the most common mental health concerns impacting collegiate student-athletes. Treatment approaches and best practices are discussed. The importance of prioritizing mental health and well-being at all levels within the university and athletics department by reducing stigma and providing access to providers is emphasized. Multidisciplinary treatment teams and coordination of care provides a holistic approach that ensures student-athletes are able to optimize their personal, social, academic, and athletic goals.

Attention-deficit/hyperactivity disorder (ADHD) is a neurodevelopmental disorder that manifests in difficulties with sustaining attention in tasks and/or hyperactivity/impulsivity. Prevalence rates vary and difficulties in objectively diagnosing ADHD may lead to overdiagnosis or underdiagnosis. Assessment should include a comprehensive evaluation, including history, physical, psychological evaluation, and questionnaires for ADHD. Stimulant medications are effective for treatment, but their use, side effects, and potential for misuse and abuse are a concern, particularly in athletes. Athletes and physicians also need to be aware of the governing body's drug policy for the sport.

Infectious mononucleosis is a common condition occurring in athletic training rooms. Most cases are due to Epstein-Barr virus infections (upward of 90%). Although treatment generally consists of symptomatic care, there is clinical variation in laboratory workup leading to diagnosis and in the method of return to play decision making. The authors suggest a systematic approach to laboratory evaluation and return to play decisions to minimize clinical variation. The most feared complication of infectious mononucleosis is potential splenic rupture. There have been several examples of the successful use of serial ultrasonography to help make maximally informed return to play decisions.

Respiratory symptoms and infections are common among athletes. Viral upper respiratory infection symptoms may precede dyspneic symptoms seen in asthmatics or worsen symptoms of exercise-induced bronchoconstriction Knowing how to instruct an athlete on use of inhalers and having an asthma action plan are critical in management of these athletes. Other life-threatening conditions that may be seen are pneumothorax and laryngeal/pharyngeal perforation. Prompt recognition and treatment are crucial if an athlete is suspected to have pulmonary compromise. Laryngeal/

pharyngeal perforations are a rare cause of issues within the training room but require a high degree of suspicion to be diagnosed and managed properly.

Athletes are susceptible to many acute illnesses that can interfere with their ability to train and compete as well as potentially affecting teammates and coaching staff. A solid understanding of the preventive measures, diagnosis, and management of such diseases is paramount in the care of an athletic population.

There are numerous disorders of the skin that occur in athletes. These include infections, mechanical injury, and inflammatory skin diseases such as dermatitis, urticaria, and others. This paper discusses some of the most common athletic skin diseases.

Athletic trainers, physical therapists, and team physicians have differing roles when providing care, yet often need to collaborate. Athletic trainers and physical therapists use a variety of therapeutic modalities and manual therapy techniques in conjunction with rehabilitation exercises to improve outcomes. Clinicians must be knowledgeable of the scientific rationale for each modality to choose the most effective treatment for the specific condition and stage of recovery. The team physician should be familiar with the use of common procedures in an athletic training room. Here, we review the most current evidence and the basic methods encountered in athletic training room settings.

# CLINICS IN SPORTS MEDICINE

**SERIES OF RELATED INTERESTED**

*Orthopedic Clinics*
*Foot and Ankle Clinics*
*Hand Clinics*
*Physical Medicine and Rehabilitation Clinics*
*Clinics in Podiatric Medicine and Surgery*

**THE CLINICS ARE AVAILABLE ONLINE!**
Access your subscription at:
www.theclinics.com

# Foreword
# Top Ten

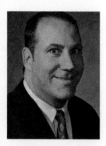

Mark D. Miller, MD
*Consulting Editor*

The Top Ten list, popularized by David Letterman in 1985, is a good way to focus on important topics. We have used this concept for lectures at the Miller Review Course for over a decade, and it has been a popular addition. It seemed only natural to adopt this approach for common primary care conditions seen by our sports medicine colleagues in the athletic training room. To pull this off, I went to my "go to" pair of primary care sports medicine physicians—Drs Siobhan Statuta and John MacKnight, team physicians for the National Champion Basketball and Lacrosse teams at The University of Virginia. As usual, they did an excellent job and assembled an expert group of fellow physicians to cover this important topic.

The articles in this issue are as diverse as the athletes who present with medical problems in the training room. This includes heart and lung conditions, concussion, traumatic and infectious injuries and illness, psychological conditions, and skin problems. In each article there is a thorough discussion of how to recognize and treat each medical condition. Hats off to the authors and editors of this issue of *Clinics in Sports Medicine*. I sincerely appreciate the job that our sports medicine primary care physicians do for our athletes across the country—we make a great team!

Mark D. Miller, MD
Division of Sports Medicine
Department of Orthopaedic Surgery
University of Virginia
James Madison University
400 Ray C. Hunt Drive, Suite 330
Charlottesville, VA 22908-0159, USA

*E-mail address:*
mdm3p@virginia.edu

Clin Sports Med 38 (2019) xi
https://doi.org/10.1016/j.csm.2019.06.008
0278-5919/19/© 2019 Published by Elsevier Inc.

**sportsmed.theclinics.com**

# Preface

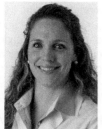
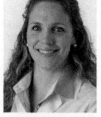

Siobhan M. Statuta, MD     John M. MacKnight, MD, FACSM
*Editors*

*I am still learning*
        *—Michelangelo*

Primary care physicians face the daily challenge of providing excellent care across a wide breadth of medical conditions in a large and diverse patient population. The specialization of "sports medicine" does little to narrow the breadth of possible conditions; to the contrary, the management of even common general medical issues superimposed on the unique demands of athletics adds additional layers of complexity. Each and every athlete must be evaluated thoroughly and with purposeful consideration of the interplay between health and athleticism within the context of their sport. Many of the intrinsic attributes of sport participation—intense physical training, contact or overuse injury risk, emotional stress, fatigue—place an athlete at increased risk to develop new medical concerns or to exacerbate underlying conditions already established. Implicitly understanding this concept allows the sports medicine provider to fully embrace the immense span of our field and to use the proper lens through which to approach and evaluate the athletic population.

With this issue of *Clinics in Sports Medicine*, our aim is to provide our readers with a concise and current review of the 10 most commonly encountered conditions seen across the general sports medicine population. As you scan through the table of contents, you will notice a range of subjects from well-known and rapidly evolving conditions, such as concussion, to less discussed but equally vital mental health considerations. We then review topics common to sports medicine practice ranging from the acute to the chronic with attention to recent updates on evaluation and management. In sum, we have produced a resource packed with valuable content ready for reading leisurely or as a bedside resource in your clinical office. We hope that you will find this issue of *Clinics in Sports Medicine* to be a trusted companion to aid you in augmenting your day-to-day sports medicine care.

This issue would not have been possible without the collaboration of several medical experts with whom it was our honor to produce this work. Thank you to all contributing

Clin Sports Med 38 (2019) xiii–xiv
https://doi.org/10.1016/j.csm.2019.06.007
0278-5919/19/© 2019 Published by Elsevier Inc.          **sportsmed.theclinics.com**

authors for your time and energy to research and create your outstanding articles. A special thanks to Dr Mark Miller for his continued support and partnership on this project. Enjoy!

Siobhan M. Statuta, MD
Departments of Family Medicine and
Physical Medicine and Rehabilitation
University of Virginia Sports Medicine
University of Virginia Health System
P.O. Box # 800729
Charlottesville, VA 22908-0729, USA

John M. MacKnight, MD, FACSM
Internal Medicine &
Orthopaedic Surgery
University of Virginia Sports Medicine
University of Virginia Health System
P.O. Box # 800671
Charlottesville, VA 22908, USA

*E-mail addresses:*
Siobhan@virginia.edu (S.M. Statuta)
Jm9m@virginia.edu (J.M. MacKnight)

# Athlete Cardiovascular Concerns in the Training Room: What Do I Do If...?

Peter N. Dean, MD[a],*, Jonathan H. Kim, MD, MSc[b],
Robert Battle, MD[c,1]

## KEYWORDS

- Cardiovascular disease • Athlete • Sports participation • Sports cardiology
- Exercise • Athletic training • Primary care

## KEY POINTS

- In general, cardiovascular concerns in athletes present to the sports medicine team through one of three portals.
  - The preparticipation examination (PPE4) is a required and self-reported history and physical that may trigger concerns because of a prior symptomatic history, family history, or a physical finding.
  - The athlete may present with symptoms or an event during training, competition, or at rest.
  - Universities, national, and professional teams with extensive resources may elect to go beyond the PPE4 with screening electrocardiograms (ECG), transthoracic echocardiograms, and/or stress testing in which the athlete may present with an incidental finding that is not accompanied by symptoms.
- Sports cardiology is a rapidly emerging discipline and sports medicine providers must collaborate with knowledgeable sports cardiology providers to ensure proper care of the athlete with cardiovascular concerns.
- Training-related cardiovascular remodeling can mimic real disease; therefore, providers must be able to separate the two. This is particularly important with incidental findings that are false positives found through screening that cannot be allowed to unnecessarily disqualify and alarm otherwise healthy athletes.

Disclosure Statement: The authors have nothing to disclose.
[a] Division of Pediatric Cardiology, Department of Pediatrics, University of Virginia, 1204 W Main Street, Charlottesville, VA 22903, USA; [b] Division of Cardiology, Emory Clinical Cardiovascular Research Institute, Emory University School of Medicine, 1462 Clifton Road NE, Suite 502, Atlanta, GA 30322, USA; [c] Division of Cardiology, University of Virginia, 1204 W Main Street, Charlottesville, VA 22903, USA
[1] Present address: 1805 Owensfield Drive, Charlottesville, VA 22901.
* Corresponding author.
E-mail address: pnd8j@virginia.edu

Clin Sports Med 38 (2019) 483–496
https://doi.org/10.1016/j.csm.2019.05.002
0278-5919/19/© 2019 Elsevier Inc. All rights reserved.
sportsmed.theclinics.com

## WHAT DO YOU DO WHEN YOUR PREPARTICIPATION EXAMINATION REVEALS A FAMILY HISTORY OF HEART DISEASE OR SUDDEN CARDIAC DEATH?

During preparticipation cardiac screening, a personal symptomatic history and a focused family history are a vital portion of the evaluation.[1,2] Importantly, in a recent retrospective survey of parents of children and young adults who had suffered a sudden cardiac arrest (SCA), Drezner and colleagues[3] found that 40% had a known family history component present before the event (most commonly family member who died of cardiac disease before 50 years of age; 27%). Many common genetic etiologies underlying sudden cardiac death in athletes, such as hypertrophic cardiomyopathy (HCM) and long QT syndrome (LQTS),[4,5] are present as a result of single gene mutations inherited in an autosomal-dominant pattern. Consequently in these cases, 50% of first-degree relatives have the disease[6] and with appropriate questioning, should be uncovered by history. We recommend exploring beyond basic questioning for "heart problems" and additionally avoiding the use of medical jargon when examining athletes. It is advantageous for the practitioner to use more basic and colloquial language in the questioning of youthful athletes. For example, asking about family members with "big or thick hearts," "enlarged or ruptured aortas," or with pacemakers or implantable cardiac defibrillators may garner clinically useful information that could otherwise be missed in the brief time set aside for cardiac screening. In addition, we advocate for basic questioning for genetically inherited valvular heart disease. Although not directly mandated in the current guidelines as part of the preparticipation screen,[7] focused questions detailing the possibility of a bicuspid aortic valve or mitral valve prolapse may be discovered that would generally be missed. Practitioners should also specifically ask about family members who passed away in unusual settings, such as single car accidents or unexplained drowning, because these could be suspicious for underlying cardiac disease.

When the family history is suspicious for a sudden cardiac event, further investigation is required. First, it is important to gather as much information about the sudden cardiac event as possible. This may require speaking with additional family members or reviewing autopsy or medical reports. Although typically not available, if genetic testing was done at the time of the sudden cardiac event, this information should be retrieved and reviewed.[8] In cases when the specific cardiac diagnosis or genetic condition is not identified, what information is available dictates what diagnostic testing should be performed from the toolkit available to the sports cardiologist. Clearly, when the diagnosis or genetic condition is identified/known, further investigation for the athlete is more focused.

Although a family history of genetic heart disease or sudden cardiac death warrants further evaluation, it is important to emphasize that this does not necessarily warrant temporary sports restriction and certainly not automatic disqualification. Decisions regarding ongoing sport and athletic participation ultimately depend on the diagnosis, disease phenotype, severity of disease in the athlete or relative, and the ability to definitively exclude heart disease in the athlete. Most importantly, as detailed later, shared decision making with the athlete, athlete's family, and other stakeholders is now recognized as an essential part of decisions for sports eligibility in athletes with underlying cardiovascular disease.[9,10]

## WHAT DO YOU DO WHEN PREPARTICIPATION EVALUATION REVEALS HEART DISEASE IN THE ATHLETE?

With improvements in the diagnosis and care of most cardiovascular conditions, athletes with heart disease have begun to embrace ongoing participation in sports and exercise. Recent data have demonstrated that some athletes with cardiovascular disease, previously deemed high risk and unsafe to continue with competitive sport participation, have had healthy outcomes without precipitated cardiac events (LQTS[11] and patients with cardiac defibrillators[12]). Moreover, the benefits of exercise on health outcomes extend to some genetic cardiomyopathies (HCM)[13,14] and complex congenital heart disease.[15,16] Within some structural and electrical cardiovascular conditions, there can also be subtle variations in phenotype that can either increase or decrease the risk of precipitating a cardiac event with sport participation. For example, patients with focal HCM, no underlying fibrosis, and no left ventricular outflow tract obstruction may be at lower risk for sudden death and therefore, after shared-decision making, be considered for sport participation (**Fig. 1**). The decision process for sports eligibility in the athlete with cardiovascular disease has evolved into a complex process. Critical appraisal of prior paternalistic practices coupled with new scientific evidence has appropriately led to a shift in paradigm to shared decision making and shared risk taking for sports eligibility.[9,10] Clinicians should be thoughtful in guiding these discussions, embrace evidenced-based practices and the lack of current knowledge, and ensure that the athlete is an integral part of the decision-making process for sports eligibility (**Fig. 2**).

Although specific recommendations exist,[17] there are certain precautions that should be put into place for any athlete with heart disease:

1. The athlete requires an evaluation from a cardiologist with expertise in the specific disease process and experience in caring for athletes. Given the complexity of most cardiac conditions and underlying exercise physiology, we recommend a multidisciplinary approach. For example, the athlete with LQTS likely requires an electrophysiologist with LQTS expertise and a general sports cardiologist. Similarly for HCM or complex congenital heart disease, experts in imaging, exercise physiology, and congenital heart disease should embrace a team approach in the care of athletes with these conditions.
2. The athlete should emphasize hydration and eating appropriate meals before competition.
3. The athlete should ensure medication compliance.
4. The athlete (ideally accompanied by an athletic trainer) should maintain scheduled follow-up appointments with physicians to assess for changes in clinical status.

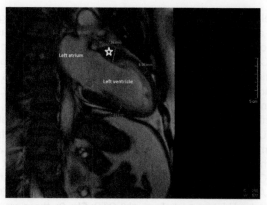

**Fig. 1.** Cardiac MRI demonstrating focal hypertrophic cardiomyopathy (*star*) with otherwise normal left ventricular wall measurements. Patient had normal left ventricular systolic function, no left ventricular outflow tract obstruction, and no late gadolinium enhancement.

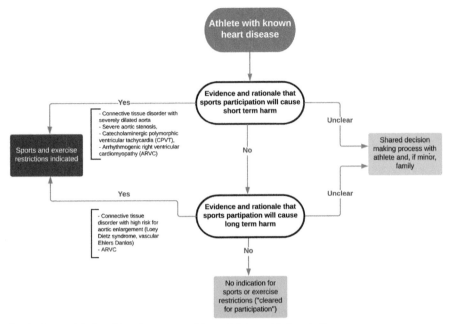

**Fig. 2.** Potential algorithm for approaching athletes with heart disease.

5. Athletic trainers and team physicians should be appropriately trained to monitor the athlete and, if needed, respond to an emergency situation. The emergency action plan (EAP) should be reviewed and practiced annually. There should be consideration of the athlete having a specific and personal automated external defibrillator (AED) on site.

These are general guidelines because individual athletes may require additional practices determined on a case-by-case basis.

## WHAT DO YOU DO WHEN YOU ARE CONSIDERING UNDERTAKING PREPARTICIPATION ELECTROCARDIOGRAM SCREENING?

Whether or not electrocardiogram (ECG) preparticipation screening should be performed in young athletes continues to be controversial and the basis of significant debate.[18–24] Although the pros and cons of athletic ECG screening and review of normal athletic ECG findings[25] are outside the scope of this review, primary care physicians and athletic trainers should be aware of the differing opinions on the topic and the pitfalls/limitations on both sides of the debate. Ultimately, it is not uncommon for a private entity (nonprofit foundation, sport organization, high school, or university) to make the determination to perform ECG screening for their athletes. The current guidelines in the United States do not mandate ECGs in the preparticipation cardiac evaluation of competitive athletes.[7] For those groups and organizations who use ECGs as part of their athlete cardiac evaluations, it is imperative that the practitioners interpreting the ECGs carry the required experience and expertise in the interpretation of athletic ECGs. Although certain conditions may be diagnosed by ECG that could be missed by the standard history and physical (LQTS; **Fig. 3**), there are many subtle athletic ECG findings that are misinterpreted as abnormal in inexperienced hands (false positive) and therefore lead to unnecessary testing and temporary sport restrictions.

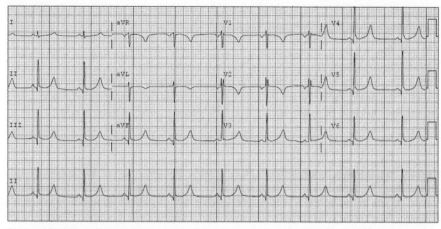

**Fig. 3.** Long QT syndrome on preparticipation ECG. Patient had been asymptomatic with no family history before presenting for university's routine athlete ECG screening. Patient subsequently had an abnormal exercise stress test (with a significantly prolonged QTc during recovery) and then underwent genetic testing, which was positive for a mutation known to cause type 1 long QT syndrome.

If preparticipation ECG screening is used as part of the standard preparticipation cardiac screen, there are several elements that should be met:

1. It is mandatory to have practitioners trained and experienced in interpretation of athletic ECGs.[26] The practitioner should be knowledgeable of recent expert recommendations (International Criteria for ECG Interpretation in Athletes[27]).
2. The program should have a method of quickly and definitively evaluating abnormal ECGs (eg, onsite or rapidly obtained echocardiogram/sports cardiology consultation). This limits extended periods of restricted time off the field, limits excess stress on the athlete and family, and decreases risk of continued participation while waiting testing (if deemed appropriate by the cardiologist).
3. It should be made clear and transparent to the athletic trainers, athletes, and families that ECGs do not exclude every form of cardiac disease. In addition, one normal cardiac screen with ECG does not exclude the possibility of a later development of structural or electrical conditions that may be acquired or genetic that evolves over time.

## WHAT DO YOU DO WHEN YOUR PHYSICAL EXAMINATION REVEALS A HEART MURMUR OR GALLOP?

Cardiac murmurs are a common finding in healthy individuals but can also be a sign of structural cardiac disease.

Benign cardiac murmurs found in healthy individuals are typically soft or "musical" systolic ejection murmurs appreciated along the left sternal border, occur early in systole, resolve with standing, and do not radiate to other areas of the body. If an athlete has a benign murmur, is asymptomatic, and has a negative family history, typically no other testing is required.

There are many types of concerning or potentially pathologic murmurs (**Table 1**). Typically, these are harsh in nature; are located anywhere on the precordium; radiate to the neck, back, or axilla; occur in diastole; or persist or worsen with standing. These types of murmurs can represent valvular heart disease (aortic stenosis, pulmonary

| Table 1 | |
|---|---|
| **Likely benign versus likely pathologic murmurs** | |
| **Likely Benign** | **Likely Pathologic** |
| Soft or "musical" in nature | Harsh in nature |
| Systolic ejection type early in systole | Holosystolic, continuous, or diastolic |
| Heard at left upper sternal border | Heard anywhere in the precordium |
| No radiation to axilla, back, or neck | Radiates to axilla, back, or neck |
| Decrease with patient standing | Persists or worsens with patient standing |

stenosis, mitral valve regurgitation), HCM (classically the murmur is caused by dynamic subaortic obstruction and worsens as the left ventricle is underfilled), septal defects or "holes in the heart" (ventricular septal defect or patient ductus arteriosus), or excessive flow through a normal heart valve (atrial septal defect or anomalous pulmonary venous return). These murmurs require an echocardiogram to diagnosis, risk stratify, dictate management, and determine sports eligibility. Other heart sounds, such as clicks or gallops, are also potentially pathologic and should be evaluated further by echocardiography. One exception is an S3 gallop, which can be normal when auscultated in a well-conditioned endurance athlete.

## WHAT DO YOU DO WHEN YOUR PHYSICAL EXAMINATION REVEALS A MARFANOID BODY HABITUS?

Marfan syndrome is an autosomal-dominant genetic connective tissue disorder that effects 1 in 5000 individuals and affects the heart, joints, bones, lungs, skin, and eyes. The cardiac manifestation is typically aortic root enlargement (**Fig. 4**), but can also be other aortic aneurysms and mitral valve prolapse. The physical findings and symptoms can be mild in childhood; meaning that some patients may not be diagnosed until high school, college, or early adulthood. The late diagnosis in athletes is evidenced by cases of sudden cardiac death and other high profile cases reported in the media.[28] The feared complication and risk of sudden death in patients with Marfan syndrome is aortic rupture and/or dissection. For athletes with tall stature, sports

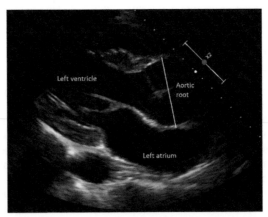

**Fig. 4.** Transthoracic echocardiogram that demonstrates a dilated aortic root on a patient with Marfan syndrome. Aortic root measures (*yellow line*) close to 5 cm.

medicine practitioners should cautiously evaluate for signs and symptoms suggestive of Marfan syndrome during the PPE4.

The diagnosis of Marfan syndrome is made using the revised Ghent criteria (**Tables 2** and **3**).[29] Although this is a complicated criteria to use in clinical practice, on-line resources are available for use when suspicion for the diagnosis is present.[30] In addition, uncovering a prior history of a spontaneous pneumothorax, ocular lens dislocation, retinal detachment, recurrent hernias, and/or unusual orthopedic injuries should raise concern and facilitate a careful investigation to exclude the diagnosis. Further testing with echocardiography and genetic testing are a part of the work-up for Marfan syndrome and should be used when clinically indicated. There are several other rare connective tissue disorders similar to Marfan syndrome, including Loeys-Dietz syndrome and Ehlers-Danlos syndrome, on the differential when the diagnosis of Marfan syndrome is considered.

## WHAT DO YOU DO WHEN AN ATHLETE HAS SYNCOPE OF UNKNOWN CAUSE DURING EXERTION?

Vasovagal syncope and orthostatic intolerance are common and typically benign in the general and athletic population. However, syncope or near syncope during exertion is less common and is a dangerous symptom that warrants a careful history, physical, and probable cardiac testing. Indeed, the presence of exertional, unheralded syncope warrants a focused cardiac evaluation in any athlete presenting with this history. In a survey of parents whose child had suffered an SCA, 30% reported that their child had near-syncope or lightheadedness, 18% had a prior episode of syncope, and 13% were also diagnosed with unexplained seizures.[3] These data underscore the importance of differentiating malignant syncope from benign syncope.

Clues for underlying benign syncope include episodes occurring at rest or with positional changes, presence of prodromal symptoms (lightheadedness, or "curtains over eyes"), no preceding cardiac symptoms (eg, chest pain or palpitations), and no family history and normal physical examination. Other key environmental factors, such as warm/humid temperatures at the time of event, episodes occurring at the finish or after finishing during recovery (discussed next), and the athlete not eating or drinking fluids before the event can suggest a more benign element to the event, particularly if the remainder of the evaluation is unremarkable and reassuring.

Red flags suggesting malignant syncope include syncope occurring during exercise, recurrent episodes, absence of prodromal symptoms (unheralded), presence

**Table 2**
**Revised Ghent criteria for diagnosis of Marfan syndrome: diagnosis of Marfan syndrome**

| Marfan Diagnosis (With no Family History) | Marfan Diagnosis (With Family History) |
|---|---|
| Dilated aortic root ($z$ score $\geq$2) and ectopia lentis | Ectopia lentis and family history of Marfan syndrome |
| Dilated aortic root and FBN1 pathologic mutation | Dilated aortic root ($z$ score $\geq$2 older than 20 years old and $\geq$3 younger than 20 years old) and family history of Marfan syndrome |
| Dilated aortic root and systemic score $\geq$7 | Systemic score $\geq$7 and family history of Marfan syndrome |
| Ectopia lentis and pathology FBN1 mutation with known aortic root dilation | |

*From* Loeys BL, Dietz HC, Braverman AC, et al. The revised Ghent nosology for the Marfan syndrome. *J Med Genet* 2010;47(7):476–485; with permission.

**Table 3**
**Revised Ghent criteria for diagnosis of Marfan syndrome: systemic score**

| Physical Examination Finding | Score |
|---|---|
| Wrist/thumb sign | Both = 3<br>Only one = 1 |
| Chest wall deformity | Pectus carinatum = 2<br>Pectus excavatum or chest asymmetry = 1 |
| Hindfoot deformity | 2<br>Plain pes planus = 1 |
| Pneumothorax | 2 |
| Dural ectasia | 2 |
| Protrusio acetabuli | 2 |
| Reduced upper segment/lower segment and increased arm/height and no severe scoliosis | 1 |
| Scoliosis or thoracolumbar kyphosis | 1 |
| Reduced elbow extension | 1 |
| Facial features (3/5) (dolichocephaly, enophthalmos, downslanting palpebral fissures, malar hypoplasia, retrognathia) | 1 |
| Skin striae | 1 |
| Myopia >3 diopters | 1 |
| Mitral valve prolapse (all types) | 1 |

*From* Loeys BL, Dietz HC, Braverman AC, et al. The revised Ghent nosology for the Marfan syndrome. *J Med Genet* 2010;47(7):476–485; with permission.

of family history of heart disease or sudden unexplained death, and if the physical examination is abnormal. In these cases, the diagnosis is pathologic until proven otherwise. If red flags are present, the recommended work-up includes:

- 12-lead ECG
- Echocardiogram
- Symptom-limited maximal exercise testing that should be tailored to the athlete specifically (ie, sprint intervals, bicycle protocols, ergometers for rowers)
- Ambulatory cardiac rhythm monitoring
- Potentially:
  - Computed tomography angiogram to evaluate coronary artery origin and course
  - MRI to evaluate coronary arteries and right and left ventricular myocardium
  - Genetic testing (as determined by data obtained from the initial work-up)
  - Implantable loop recorder (instead of more short-term Holter or event monitoring)

## WHAT DO YOU DO WHEN AN ATHLETE PASSES OUT AT THE END OF A RACE (POSTRACE BENIGN SWOON)?

In the work-up of the athlete with syncope, a common presentation is the athlete who passes out near or at the end of a race. The classic example is the athlete collapsing at the end of an endurance event and the description of feeling weak and lightheaded before the event. The athlete is able to recall the proceeding symptoms and the entire event. Because of the prodromal symptoms, there is typically lack of injury because the athlete is able to brace their body before the fall to the ground. This typically occurs at the end of the race or immediately after when the athlete has achieved maximum exercise capacity for an extended period of time.

Physiologically, the event occurs after the race because of the prior preferential shunting of blood to the muscles (for work) and skin (for conductive heat loss) along with exercise-induced reductions in systemic vascular resistance (SVR). In combination with low SVR, the athlete has low plasma volume because of dehydration related to insensible fluid losses. Once the athlete stops running, there is loss of the "musculovenous pump" that leads to lower extremity venous pooling and reduces venous return to the heart. The fall in ventricular preload, combined with low SVR and dehydration, can lead to systemic hypotension and/or bradycardia and then symptoms. Importantly, this more common presentation is easily differentiated from malignant and unheralded syncope, with the former being benign and typically without the need for a detailed work-up and temporary medical restrictions from sport participation.

## WHAT DO YOU DO WHEN AN ATHLETE COMPLAINS OF CHEST PAIN?

Although episodic chest pain at rest is generally noncardiac in origin, chest pain with exertion or exercise warrants a cardiac-specific evaluation. HCM, aortic stenosis, pulmonary hypertension, anomalous aortic origin of the coronary arteries, spontaneous coronary artery dissection, and premature coronary artery disease can all present as episodic chest pain with exercise. Specifically, HCM and aortic stenosis can manifest as exertional chest pain caused by oxygen supply/demand mismatch from left ventricular outflow tract obstruction (decreased cardiac output) and coronary ischemia (related to shorter coronary flow times with increased heart rate). Significant pulmonary hypertension negatively impacts cardiac output and there are also reports of dilated main pulmonary arteries causing coronary compression.[31] Anomalous aortic origin of the coronary artery is an important cause of sudden cardiac death in athletes[4] and must be ruled out in the evaluation of any young athlete complaining of exertional chest pain. A high index of suspicion is required for this diagnosis given the complex nature of the appropriate imaging work-up. Indeed, the gold standard diagnostic test is a coronary computed tomography angiography scan, one that is not routinely ordered among young athletic patients. Chest pain from anomalous coronary arteries is likely the consequence of the many mechanical perturbations (a slit-like orifice combined with systolic expansion of the aorta) combined with increased myocardial demand leading to ischemia. An interarterial coronary course (between the aortic and pulmonary trunk), specifically the left coronary artery arising from the right aortic cusp, is particularly high-risk and associated with sudden cardiac death.[32] Management of an anomalous right coronary origin off the left aortic cusp is much more controversial and does not always necessitate surgical repair. In a recent case from two of the authors (P.N.D. and R.B., **Fig. 5**), symptoms of chest pressure at peak exercise and an intramural course of an anomalous right coronary origin lead to surgical repair and unroofing of the anomalous vessel. Exercise stress testing has not been reliable in this population but might improve with a more rigorous exercise stress test. Although return to play guidelines after surgery remain controversial, it is recommended for at least a 3-month waiting period followed by testing to confirm no residual ischemia before resuming athletic activities.[33] Coronary artery disease is uncommon in the young athlete, but should be considered if there is a history of significant and relevant cardiac risk factors, familial hyperlipidemia, Kawasaki disease, diabetes, or a family history of early coronary artery disease.

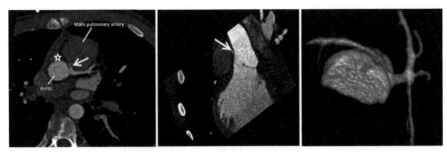

**Fig. 5.** Computed tomography scan demonstrating an anomalous coronary artery. Young athlete who presented with chest pain at peak exercise. Echocardiogram was concerning for anomalous right coronary arising from left coronary sinus. Subsequent computed tomography angiogram demonstrated the right coronary artery arising off the left coronary cusp (*yellow arrows*) instead of the right coronary cusp (*star*) and course between the aorta and main pulmonary artery. Patient underwent surgical unroofing of the anomalous coronary artery and, after reassuring testing, was able to return to sports participation.

It is not infrequent that despite appropriate cardiac testing, no diagnosis is elucidated for the cause of chest pain in the athlete. Although reassuring, these cases are frustrating to the athlete and the athlete's family. Frequent noncardiac causes of chest pain are exercise-induced bronchoconstriction, gastroesophageal reflux disease, and musculoskeletal chest pain. Venous thromboembolism/pulmonary embolism should also be considered in the appropriate clinical context or if risk factors are present (eg, family history of clotting disorders, oral contraceptives, recent immobilization from surgery).

## WHAT DO YOU DO WHEN AN ATHLETE COMPLAINTS OF PALPITATIONS/ INAPPROPRIATE TACHYCARDIA WITH EXERCISE?

Palpitations with exercise or inappropriate tachycardia with exercise also warrant further cardiac evaluation. Palpitations with exercise may represent a completely benign condition, such as orthostatic hypotension or dehydration. Other cardiac conditions that are typically benign, such as many types of supraventricular tachycardia, are also on the differential in this clinical scenario. However, some malignant cardiac conditions, such as catecholaminergic polymorphic ventricular tachycardia, Wolff-Parkinson-White syndrome with atrial fibrillation and rapid ventricular response, or ventricular tachycardia (VT) from underlying structural cardiac disease processes (eg, arrhythmogenic right ventricular cardiomyopathy), must be excluded in the work-up of exercise-induced palpitations. Clinically, the abrupt onset and termination of palpitations or inappropriate tachycardia suggest the presence of an arrhythmia, either atrial or ventricular in origin. Gradual changes in heart rate or symptoms suggest dehydration and normal sinus tachycardia. The clinical description of the onset and termination of symptoms should dictate the subsequent work-up.

Ideally, at the time of palpitations or events, a member of the athletic training staff can record a heart rate and blood pressure. Although the evidence supporting the clinical utility of smart phones and smart watches with ambulatory rhythm capabilities is limited currently, this technology may provide an alternative approach for data capture during training or competition (**Fig. 6**). Identifying the cardiac rhythm at the time of symptoms is essential in delineating the next steps in treatment.

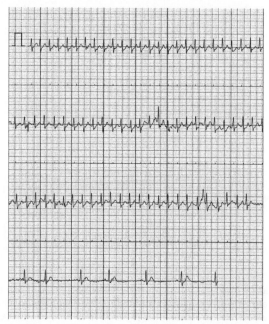

**Fig. 6.** Collegiate swimmer with sustained palpitations only during training or competition in the pool. A poolside rhythm strip from a commercially available cell phone application recorded by the athletic trainer demonstrated supraventricular tachycardia.

The work-up for these symptoms includes a baseline ECG, imaging with echocardiography and/or cardiac MRI (if arrhythmogenic right ventricular cardiomyopathy remains on the differential), and prolonged ambulatory ECG monitoring to "catch the event." Depending on specifics of the history, this may be a 24-hour ECG monitor versus a prolonged event monitor for 30 days. Typically, an exercise stress test is also necessary to attempt to elicit the exercise-induced arrhythmia. If catecholaminergic polymorphic ventricular tachycardia or VT remains on the differential, an exercise test is mandatory. If an exercise stress test is performed it is important to replicate the sports and/or activity the athlete was engaged in at the time of symptoms (**Fig. 7**). Finally, an invasive electrophysiology study may be indicated for further risk stratification of the arrhythmia or if an identified supraventricular tachycardia or VT is identified during the work-up.

## WHAT DO YOU DO WHEN AN ATHLETE SUFFERS CARDIAC ARREST (EMERGENCY ACTION PLAN)?

Even with appropriate preparticipation care, there remains risk for sudden cardiac events during sport participation. In addition to the dynamic evolving nature of many genetic cardiomyopathies, other pathologic processes exist in which SCA is the first presentation of disease. Acute processes, such as myocarditis (inflammation of the heart caused by infection) or commotio cordis, can also present with SCA. Commotio cordis occurs when a blow to the chest (eg, kick, punch, line drive from ball) occurs during a precise time period during ventricular repolarization and leads to ventricular fibrillation.[34] With myocarditis, the inflammation of the myocardium can lead to SCA when placed under stress during exercise. Survival of athletes with SCA in training or during competition is dependent on a preexisting EAP.

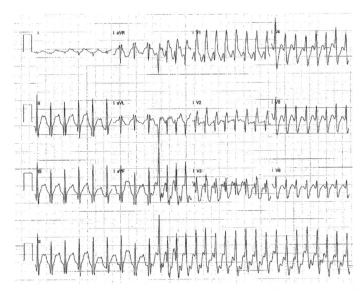

**Fig. 7.** Supraventricular tachycardia induced by exercise-specific stress test. Athlete had intermittent palpitations with exercise, so to simulate the symptoms we performed an interval sprint exercise stress test protocol. This protocol was able to induce supraventricular tachycardia in the athlete. The athlete then underwent catheter ablation and was able to return to sports participation.

The steps in the optimal design and execution of the EAP are:

1. Education and training individuals (coaches, training staff, other team members) in basic cardiac pulmonary resuscitation (CPR) and defibrillation (use of AED).
2. Having AEDs in all training facilities and sporting venues. Knowing the location of all AEDs by the athletic training and medical staff. AEDs must also have a reliable maintenance plan.
3. Quick recognition of a cardiac arrest and initiation of CPR.
4. Activation of emergency medical personnel while trained personnel use the AED on the collapsed athlete.

These steps are life-saving and have demonstrated increased survival for out-of-hospital cardiac arrests at sporting events and other areas.[35–37]

## SUMMARY

Sports medicine practitioners must be knowledgeable of the cardiac preparticipation evaluation of athletes and thoughtful when athletes present with common cardiac symptoms in the training room. Because not all causes of sudden cardiac death can be ruled out or prevented by adequate preparticipation screening, a carefully designed EAP with quick execution of CPR and defibrillation is mandatory and should be in place at all athletic events.

## REFERENCES

1. American Academy of Family Physicians AAoP, Bernhardt DT, Roberts WO, et al, editors. Preparticipation physical evaluation. 4th edition. Elk Grove Village (IL): American Academy of Pediatrics; 2010.

2. Battle RW. Sports cardiology: a discipline emerged. Clin Sports Med 2015;34(3): xv–xvi.

3. Drezner JA, Fudge J, Harmon KG, et al. Warning symptoms and family history in children and young adults with sudden cardiac arrest. J Am Board Fam Med 2012;25(4):408–15.

4. Emery MS, Kovacs RJ. Sudden cardiac death in athletes. JACC Heart Fail 2018; 6(1):30–40.

5. Peterson DF, Siebert DM, Kucera KL, et al. Etiology of sudden cardiac arrest and death in US competitive athletes: a 2-year prospective surveillance study. Clin J Sport Med 2018. [Epub ahead of print].

6. Tan BY, Judge DP. A clinical approach to a family history of sudden death. Circ Cardiovasc Genet 2012;5(6):697–705.

7. Maron BJ, Thompson PD, Ackerman MJ, et al. Recommendations and considerations related to preparticipation screening for cardiovascular abnormalities in competitive athletes: 2007 update: a scientific statement from the American Heart Association Council on Nutrition, Physical Activity, and Metabolism: endorsed by the American College of Cardiology Foundation. Circulation 2007;115(12). 1643–455.

8. Thomas MJ, Battle RW. Something old, something new: using family history and genetic testing to diagnose and manage athletes with inherited cardiovascular disease. Clin Sports Med 2015;34(3):517–37.

9. Baggish AL, Ackerman MJ, Lampert R. Competitive sport participation among athletes with heart disease: a call for a paradigm shift in decision making. Circulation 2017;136(17):1569–71.

10. Providencia R, Teixeira C, Segal OR, et al. Empowerment of athletes with cardiac disorders: a new paradigm. Europace 2018;20(8):1243–51.

11. Aziz PF, Sweeten T, Vogel RL, et al. Sports participation in genotype positive children with long QT syndrome. JACC Clin Electrophysiol 2015;1(1–2):62–70.

12. Lampert R, Olshansky B, Heidbuchel H, et al. Safety of sports for athletes with implantable cardioverter-defibrillators: long-term results of a prospective multinational registry. Circulation 2017;135(23):2310–2.

13. Pelliccia A, Lemme E, Maestrini V, et al. Does sport participation worsen the clinical course of hypertrophic cardiomyopathy? Clinical outcome of hypertrophic cardiomyopathy in athletes. Circulation 2018;137(5):531–3.

14. Sheikh N, Papadakis M, Schnell F, et al. Clinical profile of athletes with hypertrophic cardiomyopathy. Circ Cardiovasc Imaging 2015;8(7):e003454.

15. Opic P, Utens EM, Cuypers JA, et al. Sports participation in adults with congenital heart disease. Int J Cardiol 2015;187:175–82.

16. Dean PN, Gillespie CW, Greene EA, et al. Sports participation and quality of life in adolescents and young adults with congenital heart disease. Congenit Heart Dis 2015;10(2):169–79.

17. Maron BJ, Zipes DP, Kovacs RJ. Eligibility and disqualification recommendations for competitive athletes with cardiovascular abnormalities: preamble, principles, and general considerations: a scientific statement from the American Heart Association and American College of Cardiology. J Am Coll Cardiol 2015;66(21): 2343–9.

18. Sharma S. Point/Mandatory ECG screening of young competitive athletes. Heart Rhythm 2012;9(11):1896.

19. Maron BJ. Counterpoint/mandatory ECG screening of young competitive athletes. Heart Rhythm 2012;9(11):1897.

20. Lampert R. ECG screening in athletes: differing views from two sides of the Atlantic. Heart 2018;104(12):1037–43.
21. Sharma S, Millar L. Should preparticipation cardiovascular screening of athletes include ECG? Yes: screening ECG is cost-effective. Am Fam Physician 2015; 92(5):338–40.
22. Wexler R, Estes NA 3rd. Should preparticipation cardiovascular screening of athletes include ECG? No: there is not enough evidence to support including ECG in the preparticipation sports evaluation. Am Fam Physician 2015;92(5):343–4.
23. van der Wall EE. ECG screening in athletes: optional or mandatory? Neth Heart J 2015;23(7–8):353–5.
24. Harmon KG, Zigman M, Drezner JA. The effectiveness of screening history, physical exam, and ECG to detect potentially lethal cardiac disorders in athletes: a systematic review/meta-analysis. J Electrocardiol 2015;48(3):329–38.
25. Sharma S, Drezner JA, Baggish A, et al. International recommendations for electrocardiographic interpretation in athletes. J Am Coll Cardiol 2017;69(8):1057–75.
26. Prutkin JM, Drezner JA. Training and experience matter: improving athlete ECG screening, interpretation, and reproducibility. Circ Cardiovasc Qual Outcomes 2017;10(8):e003881.
27. De Vos L, De Sutter J. A comparison of the European Society of Cardiology, the Seattle and the Refined Criteria for interpreting the athlete's ECG in a preparticipation screening programme. Acta Cardiol 2016;71(6):631–7.
28. Herrick N, Davis C, Vargas L, et al. Utility of genetic testing in elite volleyball players with aortic root dilation. Med Sci Sports Exerc 2017;49(7):1293–6.
29. Loeys BL, Dietz HC, Braverman AC, et al. The revised Ghent nosology for the Marfan syndrome. J Med Genet 2010;47(7):476–85.
30. The Marfan Foundation. Available at: www.marfan.org. Accessed October 24, 2018.
31. Akbal OY, Kaymaz C, Tanboga IH, et al. Extrinsic compression of left main coronary artery by aneurysmal pulmonary artery in severe pulmonary hypertension: its correlates, clinical impact, and management strategies. Eur Heart J Cardiovasc Imaging 2018;19(11):1302–8.
32. Cheezum MK, Liberthson RR, Shah NR, et al. Anomalous aortic origin of a coronary artery from the inappropriate sinus of Valsalva. J Am Coll Cardiol 2017; 69(12):1592–608.
33. Thompson PD, Myerburg RJ, Levine BD, et al. Eligibility and disqualification recommendations for competitive athletes with cardiovascular abnormalities: task force 8: coronary artery disease: a scientific statement from the American Heart Association and American College of Cardiology. J Am Coll Cardiol 2015;66(21): 2406–11.
34. Maron BJ, Estes NA 3rd. Commotio cordis. N Engl J Med 2010;362(10):917–27.
35. Valenzuela TD, Roe DJ, Nichol G, et al. Outcomes of rapid defibrillation by security officers after cardiac arrest in casinos. N Engl J Med 2000;343(17):1206–9.
36. Page RL, Joglar JA, Kowal RC, et al. Use of automated external defibrillators by a U.S. airline. N Engl J Med 2000;343(17):1210–6.
37. Marijon E, Bougouin W, Karam N, et al. Survival from sports-related sudden cardiac arrest: in sports facilities versus outside of sports facilities. Am Heart J 2015; 170(2):339–45.e1.

# Sport-Related Concussion Evaluation and Management

Jeanne Doperak, DO[a],*, Kelley Anderson, DO[a,1], Michael Collins, PhD[b,2],
Kouros Emami, PsyD[c,3]

## KEYWORDS

- Concussion • VOMS testing • Neuropsychological testing

## KEY POINTS

- Concussion is a common issue in athletes and appropriate identification and management of the injury from the onset is key in optimal outcomes.
- The history and physical examination for a concussed patient is unique and often involves both neurocognitive testing and maneuvers specific to head injury patients.
- Concussion symptoms can be divided into specific pathways with specific treatment plans including: headache/migraine, vestibular, ocular, cognitive/fatigue, anxiety/mood, and cervical.
- Medical management of concussion including use of pharmacologic agents can become necessary when ongoing symptoms are present that affect daily activities.

## INTRODUCTION

Concussion is a challenging and often controversial medical diagnosis that can test even the most seasoned practitioner's clinical skills. Our knowledge on this topic is ever evolving. It was not so long ago that grading guidelines were based on loss of consciousness and amnesia. The medical community has seen a renaissance of discovery over the past 20 years in all areas of concussion evaluation and management. Consider that a PubMed search for "concussion" between 1990 and 2000 produced just over 1000 articles and that same search including the last 18 years expands to

Disclosure: M. Collins discloses that he is Co-developer, board member and shareholder of ImPact Applications, Inc.
[a] Department of Orthopaedic Surgery, University of Pittsburgh Medical Center, University of Pittsburgh, Pittsburgh, PA, USA; [b] Department of Orthopaedic Surgery, University of Pittsburgh Medical Center Sports Medicine Concussion Program, University of Pittsburgh Medical Center, Pittsburgh, PA, USA; [c] University of Pittsburgh Medical Center Sports Medicine Concussion Program, Pittsburgh, PA, USA
[1] Present address: 1707 Waterless Drive, Sewickley, PA 15143.
[2] Present address: 179 Mohawk Drive, Pittsburgh, PA 15228.
[3] Present address: 3345 Penn Avenue, Unit E., Pittsburgh, PA 15201.
* Corresponding author. 1052 Boomtown Lane, Latrobe, PA 15650.
*E-mail address:* Doperakjm@upmc.edu

over 10,000 publications. This article tries to capture the most recent knowledge and recommendations based on the published evidence.

## IDENTIFYING THE INJURY—FROM THE SIDELINE TO THE OFFICE

Concussion is an injury that does not discriminate, affecting all ages, gender, and level of athlete. The Center for Disease Control and Prevention estimates that between 1.6 and 3.8 million sport-related concussions (SRCs) occur annually in the United States.[1] According to the American Medical Society for Sports Medicine Position statement, 30% of all concussions in individuals between 5 and 19 years of age are sports related and result in a significant number of emergency room visits.[2] Most concussions in the United States occur in football, wrestling, girls and boys soccer, and girls basketball.[2] There are a greater number of concussions reported in games versus practice and in female athletes versus male athletes.[2]

Signs and symptoms of a concussion can range from a downed athlete unconscious on the field to a participant whose teammates and coaches notice that they are just not acting "right." In the former example, evaluation should begin with ACLS protocol and assuring airway, breathing, and circulation. A cervical spine examination should be completed and appropriate precautions taken to stabilize the patient when necessary. A Glasgow coma scale (**Table 1**) can be quickly assessed to determine if more immediate acute treatment is needed.

It is most common for a concussed athlete to present with headache and secondly dizziness.[2] Immediate onset dizziness is associated with a 6.4 times greater risk relative to any other on-field symptom in predicting a protracted recovery.[3] Other observed symptoms can be, but are not limited to, amnesia, nausea, fatigue, fogginess, difficulty concentrating, sensitivity to light and/or noise, blurred vision, and emotional lability (**Box 1**). An athlete who reports or is observed to have any of these symptoms should be withheld from play and further evaluated in a distraction-free environment when possible.[2,4]

| Table 1 Glasgow coma scale | Response | Score |
|---|---|---|
| Eye opening response | Spontaneously | 4 |
| | To Speech | 3 |
| | To pain | 2 |
| | No response | 1 |
| Best verbal response | Oriented to time, place, and person | 5 |
| | Confused | 4 |
| | Inappropriate words | 3 |
| | Incomprehensible sounds | 2 |
| | No response | 1 |
| Best motor response | Obeys commands | 6 |
| | Move to localized pain | 5 |
| | Flexion withdrawal from pain | 4 |
| | Abnormal flexion (decorticate) | 3 |
| | Abnormal extension (decerebrate) | 2 |
| | No response | 1 |
| Total score | Best response | 15 |
| | Comatose patient | 8 or less |
| | Totally unresponsive | 3 |

---

**Box 1**
**Concussion signs and symptoms**

*Signs observed:*

- Appears to be dazed or stunned
- Is confused about assignment
- Forgets plays
- Is unsure of game, score, or opponent
- Moves clumsily
- Answers questions slowly
- Loses consciousness
- Shows behavior or personality change
- Forgets events before hit (retrograde)
- Forgets events after hit (anterograde)

*Symptoms reported by athlete:*

- Headache
- Nausea
- Balance problems or dizziness
- Double or fuzzy vision
- Sensitivity to light or noise
- Feeling sluggish
- Feeling "foggy"
- Change in sleep pattern
- Concentration or memory problems

---

One of the challenges with concussion is that at times an athlete will under-report or deny symptoms to prevent being withheld from play. This requires the medical provider to have keen observational skills on the field and on the sideline. There are several sideline examination tools which help to assist the provider in correctly identifying injury such as the Sport Concussion Assessment Tool 5 (SCAT5), the Standardized Assessment of Concussion, the King-Devick test, the Balance Error Scoring System, and vestibular/ocular-motor screening (VOMS). These tests individually or combined as part of the initial sideline examination can help to provoke symptoms or physical examination signs in concussed athletes who may be under-reporting symptoms.[4] The most recent consensus statement on concussion in sport held in Berlin in 2016, and published in 2017, suggests that the SCAT5 test "represents the most well-established and rigorously developed instrument available for sideline assessment." However, the authors also go on to suggest the added utility of clinical reaction time, gait/balance assessment, video-observable signs and, oculomotor screening.[4]

As suggested above, VOMS can augment your sideline and/or office physical examination. This test, through a series of eye and head movements, stresses the oculomotor and vestibular systems and the intention is to provoke symptoms. VOMS is a brief (~5 minute) tool developed for these purposes and has shown strong consistency and the ability to differentiate between concussed and nonconcussed individuals.[3]

VOMS requires the patient to self-report the severity of their symptoms of headache, dizziness, nausea, and fogginess on a 0 to 10 scale before administration by the screener. There are 5 components: (1) smooth pursuits, (2) horizontal and vertical saccades, (3) horizontal and vertical vestibular-ocular reflex, (4) visual motion sensitivity, and (5) near point of convergence. Signs of possible vestibular dysfunction are indicated with a +2 score on any of the aforementioned symptoms following the VOMS subtests. A receded near point of convergence (eg, ocular-motor impairment) is noted if the athlete reports seeing 2 distinct images (~14-point font size) on the visual fixation stick as they slowly bring it toward their nose or when the examiner observes an exodeviation of 1 eye that measures greater than or equal to 5 cm from the tip of the nose. Please refer to **Fig. 1**, which illustrates the individual components of this examination.

As part of the initial evaluation of concussion there is no validated research supporting the need for any imaging or fluid biomarkers.[5] In addition, the commercial market has become flooded with sideline assessment tools from wearable pads to light boards, none of which has been shown to be superior to the validated tools already mentioned above.

Once an athlete has been diagnosed with a concussion, it is imperative that they are held from further participation. It is important to communicate this information to the coaching staff and, if necessary, to withhold a required piece of the athlete's equipment (ie, helmet) to assure compliance.[2,4]

## PATHOPHYSIOLOGY OF CONCUSSION

SRC is considered a mild traumatic brain injury (mTBI) resulting from biomechanical forces that are directly or indirectly transferred to the head, causing the brain to shift or move inside the skull. Subsequent changes at the neurometabolic level ensue and lead to a cascade of events at the cellular level, best characterized as an efflux of potassium and a co-occurring influx of calcium through cell membranes.[6,7] These neurometabolic changes cause the vasoconstriction of blood vessels and an overall decline in cerebral blood flow and, in turn, heighten the demand for energy (ie, glucose). Given the functional nature of this injury, it should not be of surprise that traditional imaging techniques (eg, computerized tomography) have not been successful in identifying/ diagnosing concussion but are used to rule out more severe pathology (eg, intracranial bleed or skull fracture).[4]

## IN-OFFICE CONCUSSION MANAGEMENT

SRC can lead to a constellation of symptoms that can last for months if not addressed properly.[4,8] Symptoms often manifest physically (eg, headaches/migraines, dizziness, and visual problems), cognitively (eg, attention/concentration difficulties, memory problems, and fatigue), emotionally (eg, depression and anxiety), and in other aspects of daily functioning (eg, sleep problems), with subsequent impact on the patient's ability to tolerate school, work, socialization, and athletic participation.

While during the subacute phase of the injury (1–7 days) patients often appear grossly symptomatic or "globally" impaired, there is emerging evidence suggestive of SRC being an injury that can present with independent and unique subtypes/symptom clusters.[9] These symptom profiles include: (1) posttraumatic migraine, (2) vestibular, (3) ocular, (4) cognitive/fatigue, (5) anxiety/mood, and (6) cervical. This model can provide a conceptual framework for which clinicians who manage SRC can operate and guide treatment recommendations.

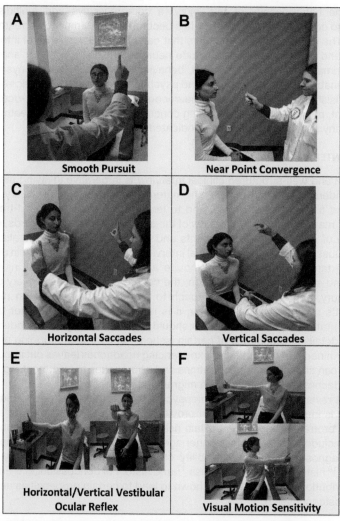

**Fig. 1.** Vestibular/ocular motor screening (VOMS) assessment. (*A*) Smooth pursuits: patient follows the examiners fingertip in a horizontal and vertical plane to a distance of 1.5 feet for 2 repetitions in each plane. (*B*) Convergence: patient focuses on a target at arm's length, which is slowly brought to the tip of the nose. The patient stops when they see 2 images of the target or the examiner notes an exophoria (outward deviation of 1 eye). Two repetitions should be performed. (*C, D*) Horizontal and vertical saccades: examiner holds fingertips 3 feet from the patient and 1.5 feet to the right and left of midline for horizontal, and 1.5 feet above and below midline for vertical. The patient moves their eyes as fast as possible from 1 fingertip to the other for 10 repetitions. (*E*) Horizontal/vertical vestibular-ocular reflex: the patient holds their thumb vertical at arm's length in front for horizontal testing and rotates their head left and right by 20° while maintaining focus on the target for 10 repetitions at a speed of 180 beats/min. The patient holds their thumb horizontal at arm's length in front for vertical testing and, in a similar manner, moves the head 20° in a vertical plane. (*F*) Visual motion sensitivity: the patient holds 1 arm in front and, while focusing on their thumb, they rotate their head and body to the left and right by 80° in 1 smooth motion at a speed of 50 beats/min for 5 repetitions (back and forth = 1 rep).

Given the heterogeneity of this injury, a comprehensive and multidisciplinary approach to concussion management has become the recommended treatment modality.[4,10] The various team of providers that can provide unique insight into concussion care and management often include neuropsychology, vestibular and exertion therapy, primary care sports medicine, behavioral neuro-optometry, physical medicine and rehabilitation, neurosurgery, and psychiatry.[11] Ideally, the in-office evaluation should consist of a clinical interview, neurocognitive testing, vestibular-ocular motor assessment, psychoeducation regarding concussion symptomology, treatment planning, and any subsequent referrals, if indicated.

## CLINICAL INTERVIEW

A thorough and well-structured clinical interview is imperative in laying the foundation for understanding the athlete, the nature and severity of the injury, to build rapport and trust with the athlete, and to lend insight into the clinical trajectories the patient may experience.[11] A review of the appropriate medical records, including integration of any sideline assessments and neuroimaging results, is also recommended. Questioning during the clinical interview should be an exercise in data gathering, with targeted questions that inquire about the mechanism of injury, acute markers and symptoms of concussion, the course of symptom recovery since the date of injury, and the general approach to treatment thus far. When discussing the patient's current symptomatology, it is not satisfactory to only get the list of symptoms; rather, the astute clinician should dig deeper to gain an understanding about the details and nuances of certain issues. For example, stopping after it has been determined that the patient is experiencing headaches leaves out important aspects that can change recommendations and approaches to treatment (eg, cervicogenic headaches vs headaches with migrainous features).

Lastly, a review of the patient's biopsychosocial history and premorbid medical conditions is imperative, as this can provide insight for the likelihood of a complicated and protracted recovery. Certain risk factors that have been identified in the literature include female sex,[12] younger age,[12] history of headache/migraine,[13] psychiatric diagnoses,[14] learning disability or attention-deficit/hyperactivity disorder (ADHD),[15,16] history of motion sickness,[17] and history of concussion.[18,19] Further, familial contributions have also been shown to lead to certain propensities and vulnerabilities postconcussion.[20]

## NEUROCOGNITIVE TESTING

Neurocognitive testing has been identified as a necessary component of concussion assessment and management, and its utility in providing an objective measure of an athlete's cognitive functioning postinjury has been well documented.[4,21] Although neuropsychological testing has been traditionally completed through paper-and-pencil formats, computerized neurocognitive tests (CNTs) have become popular with athletes for a variety of advantageous reasons. Specifically, CNTs are shorter in duration (20–30 minutes) and more logistically feasible, can be administered to multiple athletes at one time, have multiple forms with randomization for repeat administration to reduce practice effects, and provide a more accurate measure of reaction time. Further, reports are automatically generated and compared against baseline scores and previous assessments to delineate recovery and help inform decisions on return to play. There are many CNTs on the market (ie, Immediate Post-Concussion Assessment and Cognitive Testing, Automatic Neurocognitive Assessment Metrics, and CNS Vital Signs); they typically measure the domains that have been identified as being negatively affected following concussion: (a) attention/concentration,[22] (b) verbal and visual memory,[23] (c) processing speed,[24] and (d) reaction time.[24] Interpretation of scores should be done by a clinician properly trained in neuropsychological assessment and who can ensure the validity of the test data. If more extensive testing is required, a referral for a comprehensive neuropsychological evaluation can be recommended.

## VESTIBULAR/OCULAR MOTOR SCREENING

Vestibular and oculomotor dysfunction has become an increasing area of focus following concussion, given the prevalence and subsequent impact on daily functioning.[25] Therefore, it would be of importance to properly assess for these issues and their severity. Symptoms of vestibular dysfunction include dizziness, vertigo, nausea, difficulty tolerating motion, environmental sensitivities, and mental fogginess.[3,9] Common oculomotor-based symptoms include a receded near point of convergence that can lead to blurred and/or double vision, difficulties with reading and visually demanding tasks, eye pressure, and frontally based headaches.[3,9,26]

Incorporating VOMS as part of an in-office evaluation for concussion can provide the clinician with useful information regarding the role (if any) and magnitude of vestibular and ocular-motor impairment. The examination is described in detail in an earlier section above. This information can drive treatment recommendations and referrals to skilled therapies (vestibular and/or vision therapy), exercise parameters, necessary academic and work accommodations, and provide patients with knowledge as to why they are experiencing certain symptoms.

## FEEDBACK AND TREATMENT PLANNING

Proper feedback and psychoeducation has been shown to improve outcomes for certain medical conditions,[27] including concussion.[28,29] Providing feedback to the patient at the end of the evaluation should involve a review of the pathophysiology and common symptoms of concussion, discussion and implications of the neurocognitive test data, requirements for clearance to return to sport, guidelines and restrictions on permissible exercise, and review of the recommendations and referrals to treatments that are indicated. The discontinuation of self-limiting/avoidant behaviors and adherence to a regular schedule of diet, hydration, exercise, sleep, and stress management should also be emphasized at this time, to avoid exacerbating other physical symptoms. Academic and/or work accommodations can also provide assistance with a transition back to school or work in a manner that is conducive to symptom management.

## CONCUSSION CLINICAL PROFILES AND TARGETED TREATMENTS PATHWAYS

As briefly discussed earlier, the conceptualization of concussion sequelae has seen a paradigm shift to a more targeted and individualized approach that involves specific subtypes or profiles.[9,30] These profiles typically become more apparent and easier to discern after the first week of injury, when athletes often present as globally impaired. One such model that lends itself for conceptualization was first published by Collins and colleagues in 2014,[9] and includes the following 6 clinical profiles: (1) posttraumatic migraine, (2) vestibular, (3) ocular, (4) cognitive/fatigue, (5) anxiety/mood, and (6) cervical. While in some cases athletes can present with a single and clearly delineated clinical profile (eg, vestibular or oculomotor only), more often than not there is some combination that is at play (eg, vestibular, anxiety/mood, or posttraumatic migraine).[9] Therefore, it is up to the clinician to determine which of these issues is primary, secondary, and tertiary through the evaluation procedures that were discussed above. This will help develop and prioritize targeted treatment recommendations to guide patients toward a more rapid resolution of symptoms and return to play, while reducing the risk of oversight of certain issues. A brief overview of each clinical profile and its targeted treatment is given below.

### Posttraumatic Headache/Migraine

Posttraumatic headache is defined by the *International Classification of Headache Disorders, 3rd Edition (ICHD-3)*, as a headache that occurs within close temporal proximity (within 7 days) of head trauma and has the clinical features of those seen in primary headache disorders (eg, tension-type headaches and migraine).[31] They can either be acute (<3 months) or chronic (>3 months). Migraine typically presents as unilateral, pulsating, moderate to severe in intensity, and is often accompanied by photosensitivity and/or phonosensitivity and nausea/vomiting.[31] Headache has been identified as the symptom that occurs with highest frequency during the first week postinjury.[32] Patients that present with headaches may find that their symptoms are often worsened with increased stress, anxiety/mood difficulties, sleep dysregulation, and poor diet/hydration. VOMS testing will often be nonprovocative if this clinical profile is in isolation. Neurocognitive data can reflect memory (verbal and/or visual) and speed deficits.[9,13] Furthermore, patients with migraine have also been more vulnerable to protracted recovery,[13] and a familial history of migraine may also serve as a risk factor for the development of migraine symptoms following SRC.[20]

Targeted treatment recommendations for posttraumatic migraine should start with adherence to a well-regulated schedule of sleep, proper diet and hydration, exercise (eg, noncontact/nonrisk exertion), and stress management. Cardiovascular exercise that is graduated as the patient develops tolerance is often recommended.[9,11] Resuming physical activity can also provide the athlete with increased socialization and engagement in preferred activities (eg, sports), which in turn reduces stress and helps combat exacerbations of headaches/migraine. In the instance of more chronic cases, a referral for pharmacologic intervention (eg, tricyclic antidepressants) may be indicated.

### Vestibular

The vestibular clinical profile is often characterized by symptoms of dizziness, mental fogginess, nausea, difficulty tolerating complex and busy environments (eg, grocery store or school cafeteria), feelings of anxiety and panic, and a sense of detachment. Quick or sudden movements of the head will often trigger or exacerbate symptoms. Peripheral vestibular dysfunction (eg, benign paroxysmal positional vertigo) may also be indicated if symptoms of vertigo (quick and spinning sensation) are reported while rolling over in bed. VOMS testing will be the most useful tool in assessing for symptoms of a vestibular origin. The athlete may often be provoked with horizontal and/or vertical gaze stability and optokinetic sensitivity. Neurocognitive data may highlight a pattern that shows impaired processing speed and reaction time, in lieu of relatively intact memory scores. Risk factors for this clinical profile may include preexisting vestibular disorders and a personal history of car/motion sickness.[17] Furthermore, athletes who report on-field signs/symptoms of dizziness, which may indicate vestibular dysfunction, have been shown to have protracted recovery times.[33]

Targeted treatment pathways indicated for vestibular dysfunction following SRC almost always include a referral to a neuro-vestibular therapist who is trained in the nuances of these issues and can provide the athlete with an individualized set of exercises to rehabilitate these issues.[34] A structured exercise plan can also supplement and provide the athlete with certain workouts to further aid recovery. Patients with vestibular dysfunction can present with co-occurring anxiety or psychiatric symptoms.[35,36] These emotional changes have been postulated to occur as a result of the shared neuroanatomical and neuronal pathways between the vestibular and anxiety centers,[37] or as a response to the uncomfortable and panic-like sensations that can mimic vestibular symptoms.[36] In these cases, a referral for pharmacologic management to better manage the psychiatric symptomatology may be warranted.

## Ocular

The ocular-motor clinical profile is often characterized by frontally based headaches, fatigue, difficulty with visually demanding tasks (eg, reading, mathematics, and lengthy computer work), pressure behind the eyes, and difficulty with attention/concentration. Posttraumatic ocular dysfunction has been reported to be prevalent, with 1 study reporting rates as high as 69% with a group of adolescents.[26] As a result, academic and work-based performances may be negatively affected. Whereas VOMS testing may show abnormalities during smooth pursuits or horizontal/vertical saccades, a more likely finding will be a receded near point of convergence. Neurocognitive testing may reveal worsening performance on verbal memory, visual motor speed, and reaction time.[38] Risk factors for this clinical profile have been speculated to include a history of vision/ocular problems (eg, amblyopia and strabismus).

Targeted treatment for the ocular clinical profile may begin with a referral to a vestibular therapist, as they are trained to assess for and provide exercises to retrain the athlete's ocular functioning. If the athlete requires a higher level of care, an evaluation by a trained neuro-optometrist who can initiate a course of vision therapy may be indicated.[39,40] Academic- and work-based accommodation, in the form of frequent breaks when engaged in visually demanding tasks, can also be of great benefit to combat fatigue and headaches. Because patients with this clinical profile do not exhibit symptom provocation with exercise, an exertion protocol may be prescribed.

## Cognitive/Fatigue

The cognitive/fatigue clinical profile is highlighted by the exacerbation of symptoms as the day progresses. Other difficulties include nonspecific headaches that are intensified with increased cognitive effort, overall reductions in energy levels, and, at times, sleep disturbance. Difficulties with concentration in the academic or work setting may also be reported. VOMS testing in those that solely present with a cognitive/fatigue profile is often normal. However, objective neurocognitive data will indicate a global suppression of scores in the domains of processing speed, memory, and reaction time. Risk factors for this clinical profile may include a personal history of learning disability and attentional issues.[41,42]

Targeted treatment pathways for this clinical profile often include adherence to a regulated schedule of diet/hydration, exercise, and, in particular, sleep. Pharmacologic intervention is also common and has shown to be effective for symptoms associated with the cognitive/fatigue profile (eg, amantadine).[43,44] With more protracted cases, cognitive rehabilitation may be recommended; however, the research supporting this in the context of mTBI/concussion is sparse.[45] Academic and/or work accommodations can often go a long way toward managing symptoms, while at the same time not having the athlete fall behind with their responsibilities.

### Anxiety/Mood

The anxiety/mood clinical profile includes an overall increase in anxiety, ruminative thoughts, hypervigilance and hypersensitivity toward symptoms, feeling overwhelmed, sadness, and/or hopelessness. In fact, anxiety has been identified as one of the most common psychiatric manifestations of concussion.[46] Among National Collegiate Athletic Association Division I athletes, prevalence rates of anxiety have been reported as high as 73%.[47] Given these staggering numbers, it is of extreme importance to identify and determine the nature and severity of emotional difficulties following SRC, as its contribution to protracted recovery has been well documented.[48,49] Symptom report is often exaggerated with this population and sleep can be affected given the tendency for rumination and excessive worry. Periods of downtime afford opportunities for athletes to focus on symptoms, in turn exacerbating comorbid symptoms (eg, headaches). Patterns of conditioned avoidance further complicate matters as athletes can become resistant to the idea of engaging in activities/exercises that are discomforting but necessary for recovery.[35,48] Suicidal ideation should be routinely assessed for, and necessary steps to keep the athlete safe are paramount. VOMS testing may be provocative, especially with co-occurring vestibular dysfunction. Without any co-occurring symptom profiles, athletes will likely perform within normal limits on neurocognitive testing, while reporting subjective cognitive complaints. Risk factors for this clinical profile include a history of mood disorder.[14]

If vestibular symptoms are absent, athletes can be immediately started on an exertion protocol that can allow the athlete opportunities for emotional release and engagement in preferred activities. The benefits of exercise on mental health have been well established.[50] Further, strict adherence to a regulated schedule of sleep, diet/hydration, and stress management is of extreme importance. In more protracted cases, and if the degree of anxiety/mood concerns is severe and leading to self-limiting and avoidant behaviors, a referral for psychopharmacological intervention or psychotherapy may be warranted.

### Cervical

Although not directly related to cerebral involvement, the cervical clinical profile can be present in injuries with whiplash-type mechanisms.[51] Patients will often report headaches that arise from the suboccipital region of the skull and neck pain/stiffness, which are considered to be a separate entity from migraine-type headaches.[51] VOMS and neurocognitive testing do not typically show any impairment, and the athletes' report of symptoms will not reflect these issues. If this clinical profile is suspected, a referral to a certified physical therapist or a physician may be warranted to rule out any structural or ligament damage. This assessment will typically involve a range of motion (ROM) evaluation, strength test, testing of the stability of cervical ligaments, and assessment of flexibility of cervical musculature. Targeted treatments may include physical therapy with ROM exercises, soft tissue mobilization, manual cervical and thoracic mobilization, trigger point injections, and, in more protracted cases, pharmacologic intervention (eg, analgesics, anti-inflammatories, and muscle relaxants). Risk factors for this profile can include a premorbid history of cervical vulnerability.

## PHARMACOLOGIC MANAGEMENT

Concussion symptoms most often resolve on their own with time or with the appropriate physical therapies described above. However, if symptoms persist and/or inhibit participation in prescribed therapies, pharmacologic intervention can be considered. Unfortunately, strong evidence-based data do not yet exist for these treatments, so most of what is described in this section is based on anecdotal evidence.

The main areas addressed through pharmaceutical therapies are sleep difficulties, migraine, mood disorders, and cognitive fatigue. A concussion is a complex pathophysiologic process, and determining appropriate pharmacologic therapies can also be complex. One must determine which clinical profiles the patient is experiencing and, of those, which are at the core. **Table 2** summarizes several pharmacologic therapies that can be used to address these ongoing concerns. The goal of pharmacologic management should focus on the "less is more" approach, and dose adjustments should be made over time based on patient response. As you can see, several of these medications overlap and cover more than 1 concussion profile. For example, amitriptyline can be used to address difficulty falling asleep and well as migraine headaches.

When initiating pharmacologic therapy, first and foremost, sleep must be addressed. It is very hard to address symptoms if sleep is not regular. Lack of sleep can lead to or contribute to cognitive difficulties, headaches, and anxiety/depression. Proper sleep hygiene is at the core of good sleep initiation and maintenance. The goal is to achieve 7 to 9 hours of sleep each night. Sleep can also be affected by pain/headache or clinical anxiety/depression. Whatever symptom is at the root cause of sleep disorder should be targeted by the treating physician. For example, if sleep is limited by headaches but the headaches are caused by anxiety, choosing a medication that treats the anxiety would be the best first step. When insomnia is the root cause this author often starts with melatonin and reviewing sleep hygiene techniques, and only uses prescription sleep aids when conservative treatment fails.

The treating practitioner should understand that headaches can come in a variety of forms: tension, cervicogenic, chronic daily, cognitive fatigue, migraine, and posttraumatic, to name a few. A conservative approach with physical therapy, prescription or over-the-counter abortive medications, proper nutrition and hydration, stress control, and exercise should be tried before a daily medicine is added. When headaches interfere with daily life and do not resolve with the conservative measures described above, this author typically begins treatment with amitriptyline, especially in cases of associated sleep disturbance. If there is no sleep disturbance, nortriptyline can be a good

**Table 2**
**Pharmacologic treatment of concussion**

| Headache Prevention | Anxiety/Depression | Sleep Difficulties | Cognitive Fatigue |
|---|---|---|---|
| TCAs: amitriptyline/ nortriptyline (30–50 mg qd) | SSRIs: Zoloft, Lexapro, Prozac (adjust dose based on response) | Melatonin (3–5 mg) | Amantadine (100 mg at breakfast and lunch) |
| Topamax (100–200 mg qd or div bid) | SNRIs: Cymbalta (30–60 mg qd) | TCAs: amitriptyline/ nortriptyline (10–50 mg) | Stimulants: Adderall, Ritalin (5–10 mg bid) |
| Effexor (150 mg qd) | Effexor XR (75–225 mg qd) | Doxepin (10–50 mg) | Nonstimulants: Vyvanse (30 mg qam) |
| SSRIs: Zoloft, Lexapro, Prozac (adjust dose based on response) | Wellbutrin SR (150 mg bid) | Trazodone (50–100 mg) | Wellbutrin SR (200 mg qam and 100 mg qpm) |
| SNRI: Cymbalta: 30–60 mg qd | | | |
| Inderal LA (160–240 mg qd) | | | |

first-line choice. Response to treatment can be expected within 6 to 8 weeks and dosage should be maximized before abandoning one medication for another. It must be kept in mind, with so many kinds and sources of headaches, that treatment needs to be individualized and focused on the principal cause of the headache.

Cognitive symptoms can also be very frustrating for patients. They may report feeling foggy, having difficulty concentrating and focusing, or trouble with memory and processing. Cognitive symptoms can secondarily increase headache and anxieties. When cognitive symptoms dominate the symptom profile, there are several medications, many of which are stimulants, that can be helpful. Amantadine, which is not a stimulant, is a good choice to start with because it has a lower side-effect profile and still offers stimulant-like effects. It has dopaminergic properties that can help the patient feel more alert and focused, and prevent fatigue-related headaches. Amantadine has been found to improve posttest verbal memory and reaction time scores on neuropsychological testing. Stimulants, such as Adderall, Ritalin, or Vyvanse should be reserved for more severe cases of cognitive fatigue or in patients who have had a history of diagnosed ADD/ADHD. Wellbutrin is a good option if there is an underlying mood disorder associated with the cognitive complaints.

Neuropsychiatric symptoms are common in patients with prolonged recovery. If these symptoms are not addressed properly and in a timely manner, the patient can suffer from longer-term impairments. Some of the more common symptoms are anxiety, sadness, rumination about symptoms, sleep dysregulation, and hopelessness. Psychotherapy is the mainstay for mood changes/disorders, and it can be combined with a mood disorder medication when appropriate.

## SUMMARY

Treatment of concussion, especially when prolonged, needs to be a team approach involving many tools and individuals as outlined above. The information in this article is believed to be the most up to date. However, as a disclaimer, what the medical profession knows about this injury is evolving daily and it would be naive to think that, in a short time, some or even most of what we have written may be out of date. I look forward to what lies ahead in a new frontier of discovery: learning ways to continue to improve patient outcomes and prevent insult as we better understand an injury that in many ways has become an epidemic.

## REFERENCES

1. Langlois JA, Rutland-Brown W, Wald MM. The epidemiology and impact of traumatic brain injury: a brief overview. J Head Trauma Rehabil 2006;21(5):375–8.
2. Harmon KG, Drezner JA, Gammons M, et al. American Medical Society for Sports Medicine position statement: concussion in sport. Br J Sports Med 2013;47(1): 15–26.
3. Mucha A, Collins MW, Elbin R, et al. A brief vestibular/ocular motor screening (VOMS) assessment to evaluate concussions preliminary findings. Am J Sports Med 2014;42(10):2479–86.
4. McCrory P, Meeuwisse W, Dvorak J, et al. Consensus statement on concussion in sport—the 5th International Conference on Concussion in Sport held in Berlin, October 2016. Br J Sports Med 2017;51(11):838–47.
5. McCrea M, Meier T, Huber D, et al. Role of advanced neuroimaging, fluid biomarkers and genetic testing in the assessment of sport-related concussion: a systematic review. Br J Sports Med 2017;51(12):919–29.

6. Giza CC, Hovda DA. The neurometabolic cascade of concussion. J Athl Train 2001;36(3):228.

7. Giza CC, Hovda DA. The new neurometabolic cascade of concussion. Neurosurgery 2014;75(suppl_4):S24–33.

8. DiFazio M, Silverberg ND, Kirkwood MW, et al. Prolonged activity restriction after concussion: are we worsening outcomes? Clin Pediatr 2016;55(5):443–51.

9. Collins MW, Kontos AP, Reynolds E, et al. A comprehensive, targeted approach to the clinical care of athletes following sport-related concussion. Knee Surg Sports Traumatol Arthrosc 2014;22(2):235–46.

10. Resch JE, Brown CN, Schmidt J, et al. The sensitivity and specificity of clinical measures of sport concussion: three tests are better than one. BMJ Open Sport Exerc Med 2016;2(1):e000012.

11. Reynolds E, Collins MW, Mucha A, et al. Establishing a clinical service for the management of sports-related concussions. Neurosurgery 2014;75(suppl_4): S71–81.

12. Covassin T, Elbin R, Harris W, et al. The role of age and sex in symptoms, neurocognitive performance, and postural stability in athletes after concussion. Am J Sports Med 2012;40(6):1303–12.

13. Kontos AP, Elbin R, Lau B, et al. Posttraumatic migraine as a predictor of recovery and cognitive impairment after sport-related concussion. Am J Sports Med 2013; 41(7):1497–504.

14. Ponsford J, Cameron P, Fitzgerald M, et al. Predictors of postconcussive symptoms 3 months after mild traumatic brain injury. Neuropsychology 2012;26(3):304.

15. Nelson LD, Guskiewicz KM, Marshall SW, et al. Multiple self-reported concussions are more prevalent in athletes with ADHD and learning disability. Clin J Sport Med 2016;26(2):120–7.

16. Elbin R, Kontos AP, Kegel N, et al. Individual and combined effects of LD and ADHD on computerized neurocognitive concussion test performance: evidence for separate norms. Arch Clin Neuropsychol 2013;28(5):476–84.

17. Sufrinko AM, Kegel NE, Mucha A, et al. History of high motion sickness susceptibility predicts vestibular dysfunction following sport/recreation-related concussion. Clin J Sport Med 2017. https://doi.org/10.1097/JSM.0000000000000528.

18. Abrahams S, Mc Fie S, Patricios J, et al. Risk factors for sports concussion: an evidence-based systematic review. Br J Sports Med 2014;48(2):91–7.

19. Schatz P, Moser RS, Covassin T, et al. Early indicators of enduring symptoms in high school athletes with multiple previous concussions. Neurosurgery 2011; 68(6):1562–7.

20. Sufrinko A, McAllister-Deitrick J, Elbin R, et al. Family history of migraine associated with posttraumatic migraine symptoms following sport-related concussion. J Head Trauma Rehabil 2018;33(1):7–14.

21. Iverson GL, Schatz P. Advanced topics in neuropsychological assessment following sport-related concussion. Brain Inj 2015;29(2):263–75.

22. van Donkelaar P, Langan J, Rodriguez E, et al. Attentional deficits in concussion. Brain Inj 2005;19(12):1031–9.

23. McClincy MP, Lovell MR, Pardini J, et al. Recovery from sports concussion in high school and collegiate athletes. Brain Inj 2006;20(1):33–9.

24. Iverson GL, Lovell MR, Collins MW. Validity of ImPACT for measuring processing speed following sports-related concussion. J Clin Exp Neuropsychol 2005;27(6): 683–9.

25. Hoffer ME, Gottshall KR, Moore R, et al. Characterizing and treating dizziness after mild head trauma. Otol Neurotol 2004;25(2):135–8.

26. Master CL, Scheiman M, Gallaway M, et al. Vision diagnoses are common after concussion in adolescents. Clin Pediatr 2016;55(3):260–7.

27. Stewart MA. Effective physician-patient communication and health outcomes: a review. CMAJ 1995;152(9):1423.

28. Ponsford J, Willmott C, Rothwell A, et al. Impact of early intervention on outcome following mild head injury in adults. J Neurol Neurosurg Psychiatry 2002;73(3): 330–2.

29. Comper P, Bisschop SM, Carnide N, et al. A systematic review of treatments for mild traumatic brain injury. Brain Inj 2005;19(11):863–80.

30. Kontos AP, Collins MW. Concussion: a clinical profile approach to assessment and treatment. Washington, DC: American Psychological Association; 2018.

31. Headache Classification Committee of the International Headache Society (IHS). The International Classification of Headache Disorders, 3rd edition (beta version). Cephalalgia 2013;33(9):629–808.

32. Kontos AP, Elbin R, Schatz P, et al. A revised factor structure for the post-concussion symptom scale: baseline and postconcussion factors. Am J Sports Med 2012;40(10):2375–84.

33. Lau BC, Kontos AP, Collins MW, et al. Which on-field signs/symptoms predict protracted recovery from sport-related concussion among high school football players? Am J Sports Med 2011;39(11):2311–8.

34. Alsalaheen BA, Mucha A, Morris LO, et al. Vestibular rehabilitation for dizziness and balance disorders after concussion. J Neurol Phys Ther 2010;34(2):87–93.

35. Lahmann C, Henningsen P, Brandt T, et al. Psychiatric comorbidity and psychosocial impairment among patients with vertigo and dizziness. J Neurol Neurosurg Psychiatry 2015;86(3):302–8.

36. Kontos AP, Deitrick JM, Reynolds E. Mental health implications and consequences following sport-related concussion. Br J Sports Med 2016;50(3):139–40.

37. Furman J, Balaban C, Jacob R, et al. Migraine–anxiety related dizziness (MARD): a new disorder? J Neurol Neurosurg Psychiatry 2005;76:1–8.

38. Pearce KL, Sufrinko A, Lau BC, et al. Near point of convergence after a sport-related concussion measurement reliability and relationship to neurocognitive impairment and symptoms. Am J Sports Med 2015;43:3055–61.

39. Gallaway M, Scheiman M, Mitchell GL. Vision therapy for post-concussion vision disorders. Optom Vis Sci 2017;94(1):68–73.

40. Storey EP, Master SR, Lockyer JE, et al. Near point of convergence after concussion in children. Optom Vis Sci 2017;94(1):96–100.

41. Fay TB, Yeates KO, Taylor HG, et al. Cognitive reserve as a moderator of postconcussive symptoms in children with complicated and uncomplicated mild traumatic brain injury. J Int Neuropsychol Soc 2010;16(1):94–105.

42. Poysophon P, Rao AL. Neurocognitive deficits associated with ADHD in athletes: a systematic review. Sports Health 2018;10(4):317–26.

43. Reddy CC, Collins M, Lovell M, et al. Efficacy of amantadine treatment on symptoms and neurocognitive performance among adolescents following sports-related concussion. J Head Trauma Rehabil 2013;28(4):260–5.

44. Broglio SP, Collins MW, Williams RM, et al. Current and emerging rehabilitation for concussion: a review of the evidence. Clin Sports Med 2015;34(2):213–31.

45. Willer B, Leddy JJ. Management of concussion and post-concussion syndrome. Curr Treat Options Neurol 2006;8(5):415–26.

46. Iverson GL, Lange RT. Examination of "postconcussion-like" symptoms in a healthy sample. Appl Neuropsychol 2003;10(3):137–44.

47. Turner S, Langdon J, Shaver G, et al. Comparison of psychological response be-
    tween concussion and musculoskeletal injury in collegiate athletes. Sport Exerc
    Perform Psychol 2017;6(3):277.
48. Sandel N, Reynolds E, Cohen PE, et al. Anxiety and mood clinical profile following
    sport-related concussion: from risk factors to treatment. Sport Exerc Perform Psy-
    chol 2017;6(3):304.
49. Broshek DK, De Marco AP, Freeman JR. A review of post-concussion syndrome
    and psychological factors associated with concussion. Brain Inj 2015;29(2):
    228–37.
50. Penedo FJ, Dahn JR. Exercise and well-being: a review of mental and physical
    health benefits associated with physical activity. Curr Opin Psychiatry 2005;
    18(2):189–93.
51. Bogduk N, Govind J. Cervicogenic headache: an assessment of the evidence on
    clinical diagnosis, invasive tests, and treatment. Lancet Neurol 2009;8(10):
    959–68.

# Evaluation and Management of Traumatic Conditions in the Athlete

Robert Warne Fitch, MD, Jason Williams, MD*

## KEYWORDS

- Trauma • Athletic • Training • Room • HEENT • Chest • Abdomen • Primary care

## KEY POINTS

- Traumatic management of all injuries that get evaluated in the training room should initially exclude life-threatening conditions.
- Subtle injuries to the head and thorax can lead to more serious pathology and should always warrant a good history and physical examination.
- Return to play considerations can often involve many specialties for non-musculoskeletal injuries. Good communication is key with athlete, family, trainers, and physicians.
- Prevention of injury through the use of protective gear is crucial to the care of the athlete.

## INTRODUCTION

The acute on-field management of injuries is part of the scope of practice for sports medicine physicians. However, the athletic training room is often where many of the traumatic conditions that affect an athlete are diagnosed and treated. From life-threatening conditions to urgent care issues, the athletic training room will run the gamut of diagnoses. As traumatic injuries are diagnosed and managed, return to play considerations must be addressed. Communication between the athlete and multiple disciplines of medicine makes the process a combination of science and art. Our focus in this review is traumatic injuries outside of musculoskeletal injuries that are seen in the training room. The primary care sports medicine physician should be familiar with these common injuries and treatments. We present the information in a format that helps identify the condition clinically, and use evidence-based guidelines to diagnose, treat, and give return to play considerations.

Disclosure Statement: The authors have nothing to disclose.
1215 21st Avenue South STE 3200 MCE South Tower, Nashville, TN 37232, USA
* Corresponding author.
E-mail address: jaswilly@hotmail.com

Clin Sports Med 38 (2019) 513–535
https://doi.org/10.1016/j.csm.2019.06.004
sportsmed.theclinics.com
0278-5919/19/© 2019 Elsevier Inc. All rights reserved.

## HEAD, EYES, EARS, NOSE, THROAT INJURIES
### Facial Fractures

- Recent literature shows that facial fractures account for 4% to 18% of all sports-related injuries.[1,2]
- Fractures of the face require a significant amount of force and clinicians need a high level of suspicion for life-threatening injuries that require immediate interventions.

### Orbital fractures
**Etiology/incidence**

- Any of the 6 bones (frontal, maxillary, zygomatic, lacrimal, sphenoid, ethmoid) that comprise the orbit can be involved in orbital fractures. The most common orbital fracture involves the orbital zygomatic region and will commonly result in orbital floor fractures.[3] Patients often present following blunt trauma. Forces directed over the orbit can get transferred in a buckling manner, resulting in fractures across the orbital walls.

**Clinical examination**

- Clinical examination findings often include enophthalmos with periorbital ecchymosis and relative ptosis. Restricted upward gaze, diplopia, and infraorbital hypethesia should alert the clinician to entrapment of muscles and nerves into fracture segment. Other injuries to varying structures including globe injuries need to be assessed. Injuries involving nerves or rectus muscles may elicit parasympathetic responses (nausea, pain, dizziness) during extraocular testing.

**Workup**

- This will mostly focus on imaging with noncontrast computed tomography (CT) of orbits/maxilla. Thin slice coronal images give the best view of these fractures. Büttner and colleagues[4,5] found that of 1676 patients with head injury and 1 or 2 black eyes, 68% had some type of orbital fracture on CT. They recommend that all minor head trauma with orbital ecchymosis obtain CT imaging.

**Treatment**

- Treatment in the training room will focus on avoiding blowing the nose or performing any type of Valsalva maneuver. Antibiotics can be considered, as some injuries have facial lacerations and can be considered open fractures. Ice and other conservative measures are always important. Urgent surgical therapy may be needed when visual changes related to nerve or ocular muscle entrapment or enophthalmos is present.

**Return to play**

- There is no good evidence on when to return to sport, but classic teaching is 6 weeks for noncontact sports and 3 months for combat sports. Custom face shields may be helpful in some cases, although return to sport decisions should be agreed on by ophthalmology and facial surgery.

### Mandible fractures
**Etiology/incidence**

- Condyle fractures are the most common site in mandible fractures and are seen 20% to 40% of the time. The "U" shape of the mandible lends fractures to often occur to bilateral condyles. Symphyseal fractures often may be missed on Panorex imaging.

## Clinical examination

- Athletes will have pain and swelling at the site of the fracture. Direct palpation and checking for facial asymmetry is important and accounting for missing teeth is paramount. Malocclusion, along with palpable and visible step offs may be present. The *tongue blade test*, in which the athlete bites down on a tongue blade while the clinician rotates it, can be used. If the patient is able to break the tongue blade by biting down on it while it is rotated, there is a 95% negative predictive value of no fracture.[6] Commonly there are lacerations and intraoral injuries and open fracture treatment must be considered (**Fig. 1**).

## Workup

- Panorex and maxillofacial CT scans can be used to identify fractures.

## Treatment

- Initial injury stabilization can be done with an elastic wrap. Nondisplaced fractures can be treated conservatively with analgesia and liquid diet with early follow-up (1–2 weeks). Surgical intervention is needed with malocclusion or displaced fractures. Wiring of the jaw leaves it immobilized for approximately 4 to 6 weeks.

## Return to play

- Return to noncontact sport can be seen in 4 to 6 weeks but contact sports may be delayed 2 to 3 months.

### *Midface fractures*
### Etiology/incidence

- Midface fractures occur due to direct impact. The zygoma is second to the nasal bone as most commonly injured because of the lower forces required to fracture this bone. Leforte, in the 1900s, classically described maxillary fractures as 1 of 3 categories based on the superior level of the fracture line:
  - Leforte I: horizontal fracture of maxilla above the root apices and below the nose (**Fig. 2**)
  - Leforte II: transverse fracture through nasal bones, infraorbital rim, and proceeds laterally through the maxilla
  - Leforte III: "craniofacial dysfunction," where the midface separates from cranial base

## Clinical examination

- The examination of midface injuries may reveal flattening, asymmetry of the midface, epistaxis, malocclusion, dental injuries, subconjunctival hemorrhage,

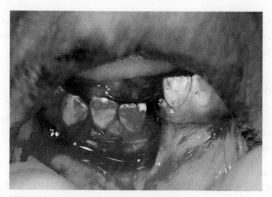

**Fig. 1.** Open mandible fracture after direct blow to face with baseball. (*Courtesy of* Lawrence Stack, MD, Nashville, TN.)

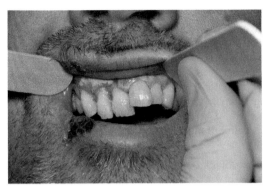

**Fig. 2.** Type 1 Leforte fracture of midface (fracture line above tooth root apices). (*Courtesy of* Lawrence Stack, MD, Nashville, TN.)

diplopia, ecchymosis, and paresthesia (infraorbital nerve). Midface instability should alert clinicians to the presence of Leforte injuries.

**Workup**
- Most of these injuries must be evaluated by CT imaging, as it provides more detail. Three-dimensional reconstructions can help with surgical planning

**Treatment**
- Injuries to the midface can be very serious, and evaluation must include assessing the airway and the remainders of the ABCs (airway, breathing, circulation). If the athlete is otherwise stable, a forward-sitting positioning can help with mouth breathing and allow blood to drain. Most midface fractures are treated with open reduction and fixation to restore any cosmetic deformity and return function. Prophylactic antibiotics are useful because of the high likelihood of open fracture. Isolated zygomatic fractures with minimal displacement may be treated conservatively or delayed to assess for deformity once the swelling subsides.

**Return to play**
- Return to play is widely varied. Common practice is to return to sport at approximately 6 weeks, with noncontact sports returning sooner. Exceptions to these rules apply to combat sports in which 3 months has been recommended for return.[7,8]

*Eye Trauma*

Blunt trauma is the leading cause of serious eye injury. Polycarbonate lenses should meet American Society of Testing and Materials standards for protection, which can significantly reduce risk.

*Ruptured globe*
**Etiology and incidence**
- Occurs in any full-thickness injury to sclera or cornea and is an ophthalmologic emergency requiring treatment by an ophthalmologist. Predictors of a poor outcome include an initial visual acuity of just light perception or no light as well as wounds larger than 10 mm.[9]

**Clinical examination**
- Without exerting too much pressure on the globe, a careful and systematic approach should be taken to evaluate the eye because subtle findings can still be a rupture (**Fig. 3**). The importance of documenting initial visual acuity

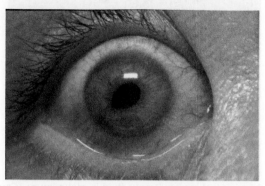

**Fig. 3.** Very subtle open globe injury with noted irregular pupil. (*Courtesy of* Lawrence Stack, MD, Nashville, TN.)

assessment is key. Looking for uveal tissue protrusion, irregular pupils, and lacerations of the cornea are important clues. "Siedel sign" is the leaking of vitreous fluid seen under black light after fluorescein staining (**Fig. 4**). A hyphema, or blood in the anterior chamber, may be present.

## Workup
- Nothing should delay prompt ophthalmologic evaluation. CT imaging can help identify subtle globe trauma.

## Treatment
- The initial management in the training room should focus on shielding the eye and leaving/securing any foreign object in place. A Styrofoam cup is a great tool for this. Tetanus status will need to be updated and prophylactic antibiotics should be considered. Analgesia and antiemetics will help prevent Valsalva-related pain and nausea. Definitive treatment is surgical.

## Return to play
- There are no specific evidence-based guidelines available. Risks and benefits of participation should be in consult with ophthalmology.

## *Corneal abrasions*
### Etiology/incidence
- An injury that occurs to the most anterior layer of the eye, corneal abrasions account for more than 10% of all ocular injuries in the National Basketball Association.[10] Fingers and balls are the usual culprits, but wearers of contact lenses are also susceptible.

### Clinical examination
- A red and injected eye with tearing and photophobia is common as well as a foreign body sensation and worsening symptoms with blinking or rubbing. Fluorescein staining will produce a yellow-green injury pattern on blue background (**Figs. 5** and **6**). Visual acuity is often normal, but may be affected because of pain, tearing, and position of the abrasion. Eversion of the upper and lower lids is an important portion of the examination when looking for any foreign body.

### Workup
- This is classically diagnosed via clinical examination, which can be greatly helped by the use of a slit lamp. Fluorescein is important in looking for abrasions and to differentiate a more serious globe injury (Seidel sign).

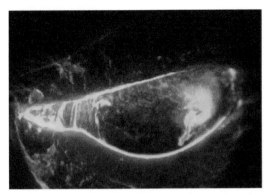

**Fig. 4.** Siedel sign showing leaking of vitreous fluid in globe injury. (*Courtesy of* Lawrence Stack, MD, Nashville, TN.)

### Treatment

- Treatment focuses on pain control. Eye patches are not recommended. Topical antibiotics are often used as prophylaxis and the practitioner must consider anti-Pseudomonal treatment in contact lens–induced injury. Tetracaine may be used to help facilitate an examination but also helps with acute pain control. Classic teaching has warned against outpatient use of topical anesthetics as it can interfere with corneal epithelialization. However, recent studies and reviews in emergency medicine literature have shown that dilute topical anesthetics for a short course as well as use of Tetracaine for 24 hours does not delay healing.[11]

### Return to play

- Uncomplicated corneal abrasions heal within 24 to 72 hours and these patients should follow-up with an ophthalmologist to document wound healing. Return to play is guided by a decrease in symptoms and may require short-term eye protection.

### Retinal hemorrhage and detachment
### Etiology/incidence

- Direct trauma to the globe/orbit can transmit forces to the retinal surface leading to injury. Violent exercises that produce strong Valsalva have also been reported to cause retinal detachment.

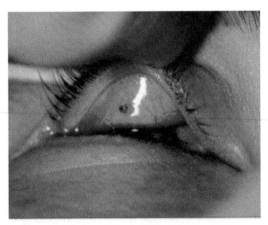

**Fig. 5.** Embedded foreign body in upper eyelid causing corneal abrasion. (*Courtesy of* Lawrence Stack, MD, Nashville, TN.)

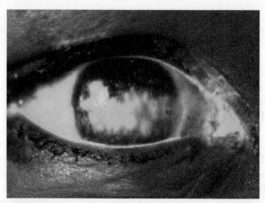

**Fig. 6.** Corneal abrasion seen under blue light after fluorescein staining. (*Courtesy of* Lawrence Stack, MD, Nashville, TN.)

### Clinical examination

- Patients describe many forms of visual floaters. Visual acuity may be affected if detachment involves the macula.

### Workup

- Patients will need a dilated eye examination. Multiple studies have indicated that ocular ultrasound exhibits good diagnostic accuracy as well.[12]

### Treatment

- Referral to the emergency department is important, as surgical evaluation and intervention are common. Depending on the acuity of visual symptoms/loss determines timing of surgery.

### Return to play

- Return to play is guided by the location of detachment and its effect on central vision. Return to play should be determined in consultation with eye/retina specialist.

## Nasal Trauma

### Epistaxis
#### Etiology/incidence

- Acute epistaxis is commonly associated with many kinds of trauma to the face. Ninety percent of nose bleeds are anterior from the Kiesselbach plexus. Posterior bleeds can be difficult to control and will likely need emergency department referral and otolaryngology (ENT) evaluation.

### Clinical examination

- Acute injuries need hemorrhage control to visualize the source of bleeding. If the patient is able to blow his or her nose to remove clots, then the examiner may achieve a better visualization. A nasal speculum can also aid in locating the source of bleeding. It is important to document the examination of other areas of injury around the face when related to trauma.

### Workup

- An isolated, controlled epistaxis needs no further workup, but in setting of trauma, a CT scan will assist to rule out fractures.

### Treatment

- Initial treatment on the sideline includes having the athlete blow each nostril, then hold compression for up to 15 minutes with a head-forward position to avoid blood from pooling in the posterior pharynx. Ice to back of head/neck can also help decrease vagal tone, thereby allowing bleeding to slow and help the clotting process.

○ Silver nitrate cautery is an option if the source is visualized.

○ Consider use of a vasoconstrictive solution, such as Afrin or lidocaine with epinephrine.

○ Nasal tampon devices are effective in bleeding that cannot be visualized or controlled. Before insertion, they can be soaked in a vasoconstrictive solution and placed along floor of the nasal cavity. Packing may need to be maintained for 24 to 48 hours to allow for clot formation. In this case, broad-spectrum antibiotic coverage especially for *Staphylococcus aureus* is important.

○ Posterior bleeding can be controlled with a double balloon device or Foley catheter if available. An immediate emergency department referral is needed for a more detailed ENT evaluation.

**Return to play**

- If nasal packing is needed for hemorrhage control, this should restrict return. An athlete whose bleeding has stopped with a simple gauze or compression and no other serious injury may be considered safe to return.

*Oral Trauma*

*Dental injuries*
**Etiology/incidence**

- Two distinct populations need consideration in cases of oral trauma, adults and children, because of the presence of primary teeth in children. Children have more pulp, thus more fractures occur through pulp. Adults have more dentin, which makes fractures through pulp less likely.[13] The Ellis Classification system is used to categorize fractures.

**Clinical examination**

- The athlete's tooth needs to be evaluated for fractures, laxity, and soft tissue injuries. Missing teeth will need thorough evaluation of where they may have gone and aspiration is always a concern. It is also important to recognize traumatic displacement or luxation. Dental trauma can range from a mild concussion (pain to palpation of tooth without mobility) to intrusion or complete avulsions.

**Workup**

- The clinical examination is usually more than adequate, but if there is concern for other facial injury, a panoramic radiograph and CT of facial bones are studies of choice.

**Treatment**

- A displaced or avulsed primary tooth should not be replaced or manipulated and the athlete should seek dental evaluation urgently. Children should stay on a soft or liquid diet and be provided adequate analgesia.

- Fracture management involves recognizing the class of injury.
  ○ Ellis 1 fractures are painless injuries to the enamel and may be referred to dentistry for cosmesis.
  ○ Ellis 2 fractures involve the dentin and are quite sensitive and painful. The clinician should cover the tooth with dental cement and refer to a dentist within 24 hours.
  ○ Ellis 3 fractures extend into the pulp, and often a reddish hue can be seen in fracture segment. These injuries are painful and have an increased risk of

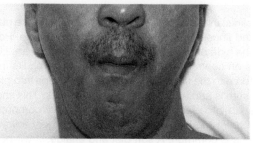

**Fig. 7.** Bilateral dislocations of mandible causing underbite appearance. (*Courtesy of* Lawrence Stack, MD, Nashville, TN.)

infection. Covering the fracture with cement or bone wax and immediate referral to a dentist is warranted.

- A dental avulsion of a permanent tooth should be reimplanted as soon as possible. The tooth may be rinsed with saline and placed in milk, saline, or Hank's solution for transport to the dentist. Tooth survival depends on delicate periodontal ligament cells. A splint should be applied with the use of suture or a commercially available device. Skin glue along with thin, wirelike, bendable metal have been used in the emergency department to splint a tooth to adjacent teeth.
- Dental luxation will need dental evaluation depending on the extent of injury.

### Return to play
- Return to sport depends on the extent of injury and bleeding control. Prevention is paramount with the use of mouth-guards.

## Mandible dislocation
### Etiology/incidence
- Inciting events can be direct trauma or a simple yawn. Mandibles most commonly displace anteriorly in which the condyles sit anterior to the eminence of the temporal bone. Posterior dislocations have been reported whereby the condyle gets pushed toward the mastoid with direct trauma. Auditory canal injuries can be seen in this case as well.

### Clinical examination
- Malocclusion is the hallmark of a mandibular dislocation. Bilateral dislocations result in an under-bite–type of appearance (**Fig. 7**). A palpable depression can be felt near the temporomandibular joint. The "tongue blade test" can be used to aid in examination. Evaluation of the ear canals is important to look for lacerations and open fractures.

### Workup
- Diagnosis may be made from the examination, but trauma can result in mandibular fracture best seen on radiograph or CT or imaging.

### Treatment
- Prompt management will aid in reduction before the masseter and pterygoid muscles start to spasm and make the relocation more difficult. A common method of reduction of anterior dislocations is to place the clinician's thumbs at the back of the athlete's lower molars intraorally and exert downward and posterior pressure to get condyles back into temporal groove. It is important to place some rolled gauze or padding on the thumbs, as reduction can cause the jaw to close and bite down on the clinician's thumbs. Another extraoral approach is that

in which the clinician stands in front of patient, thumbs are placed over mandibular ramus, and fingers behind the angle of the mandible. Posterior pressure is placed over the side of dislocation with the thumb and an anterior pulling force by the fingers on contralateral side. This technique results in a type of twisting or rotational force to the mandible. Once one side slips into place, then posterior directed pressure is applied over the opposite cheek. This should allow the second side to snap into place. A soft cervical collar or compression wrap can be used to then splint the jaw. Oral maxillofacial surgery follow-up is imperative, as reoccurrence is common. A soft diet and analgesia will help in recovery.

**Return to play**
- No specific guidelines exist. Reduction and pain control should allow for return.

## Neck Trauma

Traumatic neck injuries in sports can be catastrophic because of vital structures within this region, and may require prompt management on the field. Cervical spine injuries are common; however, serious spinal cord injury is rare.[14]

- Other vital structures of the neck, such as the airway or blood vessels, that suffer trauma are likely to need emergent, on-site management as well as transport to the emergency department.

### Stingers
**Etiology/incidence**
- More than 50% of college football players experience a stinger in their 4-year career. There are 3 proposed mechanisms of injury:
  - Direct compression of brachial plexus.
  - Traction injury to the brachial plexus.
  - Cervical nerve root compression caused by hyperextension of neck.

**Clinical examination**
- A stinger, by definition, is a unilateral injury to the brachial plexus that causes transient, unilateral neurologic symptoms to 1 arm that resolves in a short time. Bilateral symptoms are worrisome for spinal cord problems and require additional workup and imaging. Numbness, tingling, and weakness have all been described, but should be unilateral and resolve in seconds to a few minutes.

**Workup**
- Athletes should be assessed for midline neck pain, pain with range of motion to the neck, and bilateral sensory and strength deficits. True stingers do not require any imaging or additional workup, as the athlete's symptoms should resolve quickly. Bilateral symptoms are spinal cord injuries until proven otherwise and require emergent stabilization and evaluation with imaging including MRI.

**Treatment**
- Acute stingers resolve spontaneously and quickly. Prevention of cervical stretch and plexus compression can be helped with neck roll or pads. Some advocate that 3 or more stingers in a season require further neurologic evaluation.[15]

**Return to play**
- Once there is symptom resolution and strength has returned to normal, the athlete is cleared to play.

## CHEST INJURIES

Although the overall incidence of chest trauma in sports is rare, team physicians must be knowledgeable of potential injuries and be thorough in their evaluations. Although most injures may be simple contusions or strains (50%), life-threatening injuries can occur that require emergent referral and treatment. Initial on-field and training room evaluation should follow the basic principles of injury evaluation outlined in Advanced Trauma Life Support (ATLS), focusing on airway, breathing, and circulation. These injuries frequently require advanced imaging and diagnostic workups.[16,17] Although rare, these injuries can result in prolonged absence from play, with 1 recent study finding that only 42% of athletes with chest trauma returned to sport within 1 week from injury.[17]

### *Rib Fracture*

#### *Etiology and incidence*

- Rib fracture is a common result of chest trauma related to a direct blow to the thorax.

#### *Clinical examination*

- Athletes will complain of chest pain with respiration and have focal pain on direct palpation of the ribs. Many fractures occur laterally, and the examiner may elicit lateral rib pain, if a fracture is present, by simultaneously compressing the anterior sternum and posterior spine with the palms of their hands.

#### *Workup*

- Posteroanterior and lateral chest radiographs and/or rib series can be performed. Ultrasound (looking for cortical irregularity) and CT scans have both shown higher sensitivities and can be performed if radiographs are negative yet suspicion remains.[18,19]

#### *Treatment*

- It is important to consider and rule out additional injuries (pneumothorax, kidney, liver, spleen).
- Supportive care with nonsteroidal anti-inflammatory drugs, acetaminophen (Tylenol), or nerve blocks may be necessary. Splinting with tape also may be helpful.

#### *Return to play*

- Depending on the sport, contact activity should be guarded/limited for the first 2 to 3 weeks with consideration of a rib protector for 6 to 8 weeks.[20]

### *Pulmonary Contusion*

#### *Etiology and incidence*

- Rare, but can occur with direct blunt trauma and rapid deceleration injuries to the thorax.[21,22]

#### *Clinical examination*

- The presentation varies and may be delayed. Clinical symptoms may be vague, including pleurisy, persistent shortness of breath, hypoxia, hemoptysis, and tachypnea. Auscultation may reveal crackles or wheezing, although examination may be normal.[16]

*Workup*

- Initial chest radiographs may be normal, as contusions/infiltrates may not develop for 4 to 48 hours after injury. CT scan imaging is considered the gold standard and will show early findings immediately (**Fig. 8**).[23]

*Treatment*

- Supportive care with analgesics and supplemental oxygen as needed.

*Return to play*

- Based on resolution of symptoms and normalization of chest radiograph. Most resolve within 1 to 2 weeks.[20,24]

## Pneumothorax/Tension Pneumothorax

*Etiology and incidence*

- A pneumothorax occurs when air becomes trapped between the visceral pleura of the lung and the chest wall. These can occur spontaneously or from a direct blow to the chest. Spontaneous pneumothoracies most often occur in tall, thin male individuals and may be associated with forceful coughing, weightlifting, or running.[25] A traumatic pneumothorax can occur from blunt trauma to the chest and may be associated with rib fractures. A tension pneumothorax is an acute life-threatening emergency that develops when a 1-way valve air leak develops and air is forced into the thoracic cavity without means of escape. The increased pressure due to entrapped air can displace the mediastinum, decreasing venous return and cardiac function. This compresses the opposite lung and can cause cardiopulmonary arrest.[26]

*Clinical examination*

- Patients may complain of chest pain and shortness of breath. Auscultation may reveal decreased breath sounds or hyperresonant lung fields with percussion, although clinical examination is only 50% sensitive. Patients with tension

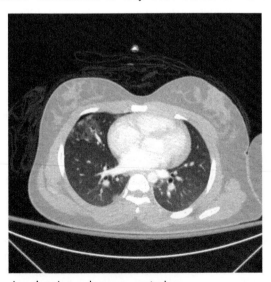

**Fig. 8.** CT scan imaging showing pulmonary contusion.

pneumothorax will present in severe distress with decreased or absent lung sounds, distended neck veins, tracheal deviation away from the side of injury, hypoxia, tachypnea, tachycardia, and hypotension.

## Workup

- Chest radiographs are historically the first study obtained (**Fig. 9**). Sensitivity may increase with images taken during exhalation.[27] Point of care ultrasound has become increasingly used on the field and in the training room with sensitivities and specificities reported better than radiographs.[28,29] Ultrasound will show lack of normal lung sliding in patients with a pneumothorax. The "sandy shore" sign is described when looking at a normal lung with M mode (**Figs. 10** and **11**). CT scan imaging is still the gold standard and should be done when the diagnosis is in question.
- For patients in whom there exists a high level of suspicion for a tension pneumothorax and who have respiratory and/or cardiovascular compromise, emergent treatment should be performed if imaging will cause any delay in definitive care.

## Treatment

- If the patient is stable and the pneumothorax is small (less than 20% lung involvement), observation may be sufficient. Pneumothoraces reabsorb at a rate of 1.25% per day. Most patients should be admitted with serial chest radiographs, and given supplemental oxygen, which increases the absorption rate threefold.[27,30]
- Small tube thoracostomy may be indicated in larger pneumothoraces or in unstable patients to expedite healing.
- A tension pneumothorax in an unstable patient should be immediately treated with needle decompression at the second intercostal space, mid-clavicular line on the side of injury, and/or acute chest tube placement, nipple level, fifth intercostal space mid-axillary line.[26]
- Serial imaging with chest radiographs will confirm resolution and healing of pneumothorax.

## Return to play

- Athletes should be withheld from play until complete resolution of the pneumothorax is seen on chest radiograph.

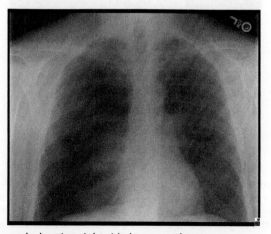

**Fig. 9.** Chest radiograph showing right-sided pneumothorax.

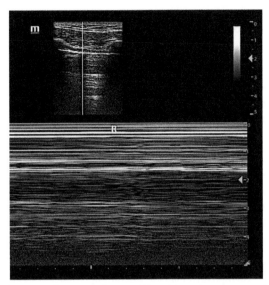

**Fig. 10.** Ultrasound image of pneumothorax. Using M mode, a pneumothorax shows linear lines below the pleural line because no expanded lung tissue is present to create echo (stratosphere sign or barcode sign).

- Athletes should not be allowed to fly for 2 weeks after complete resolution due to increased risk of worsening the pneumothorax. As pressure decreases at altitude, volume of gas increases and pneumothoracies may increase 25%.[31]

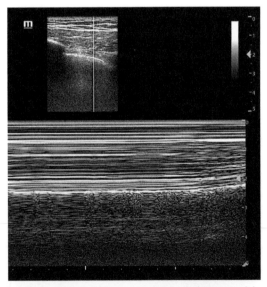

**Fig. 11.** Ultrasound image of normal lung. Using M mode, normal lung shows granular appearance below pleural line (sandy beach sign). Tissue above the chest wall that does not move is linear in appearance. As normal lung inflates with breathing, the motion of the lung changes the brightness of the echoes that return to the machine, creating a granular appearance.

## *Sternoclavicular Dislocation*

### *Etiology and incidence*

- Rare, reported to be involved in fewer than 5% of shoulder injuries.[32] Typically caused by a direct blow to the chest wall or by falling on the lateral aspect of a shoulder. Anterior is more common than posterior dislocations, although posterior dislocations have a much higher associated injury risk due to compression of the mediastinal structures.

### *Clinical examination*

- Patients will have deformity, swelling and pain on palpation of the sternoclavicular (SC) joint.

### *Workup*

- A serendipity view anteroposterior radiograph with beam shot at a 45-degree angle cranially can be helpful, although CT scan is study of choice (**Fig. 12**).

### *Treatment*

- Anterior dislocations can often be treated conservatively/nonoperatively. Posterior dislocations should not be reduced in the training room or emergency department. These should be taken to the operating room for reduction open versus closed by orthopedic surgeons with thoracic/vascular surgery present as backup in case there are injuries to the underlying mediastinal structures that decompensate after reduction relieves pressure.[32]

### *Return to play*

- Varies depending on symptomatology. Full return may take 4 to 6 weeks after reduction. The athlete should have no further symptoms of pain or instability on examination.[20]

## ABDOMINAL INJURIES

Abdominal injuries in sports are rare, however, sports participation does account for 10% of all abdominal injuries; second-most after car accidents.[33] The lower ribs offer some protection, yet the abdomen is largely unprotected placing athletes at risk. Direct trauma can occur in collision and contact sports (football, soccer, hockey) as well as high-velocity sports due to speed and falls (eg, cycling, gymnastics, skiing). Trauma can also occur from ball and stick impact from baseball and lacrosse. Although infrequent, life-threatening scenarios can develop and immediate identification and treatment should be initiated. Although sports medicine physicians may not provide definitive treatment, medical staff should be familiar with common traumatic injuries encountered on the field, as well as workup, treatment options, and return to play criteria.

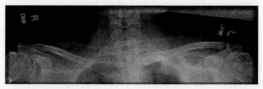

**Fig. 12.** Serendipity view showing left anterior sternoclavicular joint displacement.

### Rectus Sheath Hematoma

#### Etiology and incidence

- Caused by a direct blow resulting in bleeding into the musculature from injury to epigastric veins or artery.

#### Clinical examination

- Patients will present with bruising/hematoma over the rectus abdominus musculature with focal pain on palpation of hematoma site.

#### Workup

- Patients typically have pain with sit-ups and improvement with hips flexed. The pain should be localized to the rectus sheath. The affected athlete will have pain with flexing the abdominal musculature ("Carnett sign") but should not have peritoneal signs or severe pain on palpation elsewhere in the abdomen.[34] Ultrasound can show the hematoma with sensitivities ranging from 30% to 100%[35]; however, CT is the gold standard imaging modality and can show additional injuries if concerned.

#### Treatment

- Most will self-tamponade. Rest, ice, and compression may be helpful. In rare cases, surgical evacuation and ligation may be necessary.

#### Return to play

- Athletes may return to play once the pain and symptoms have resolved (typically 1–2 weeks). Padding to protect from repeat injury should be considered.[36]

### Liver

#### Etiology and incidence

- The liver is the most frequently injured abdominal organ in all traumas and the third most frequently injured in athletics.[37] Injury can occur from a direct blow causing a crush injury with subcapsular and intraparenchymal hematomas or from deceleration injuries with laceration to the thin capsule and underlying attached parenchyma as it continues to move.

#### Clinical examination

- Patients will have persistent and often worsening pain with palpation of the right upper quadrant commonly with radicular pain to right shoulder ("Kehr sign"). Vital signs are initially normal in 50% of patients, so repeat examinations and reassessment are critical to accurately diagnose. Tachycardia and hypotension may be late findings.[38] Serial painful abdominal examinations or the presence of peritoneal signs should prompt definitive imaging.

#### Workup

- A Focused Assessment with Sonography in Trauma (FAST) examination looking for free fluid can be helpful with 85% sensitivity reported, although CT scan remains the gold standard in diagnosis.[39] Laboratory tests, including liver function tests, should be obtained.

*Treatment*

- Patients be should admitted for observation. Liver injuries are graded 1 to 5 based on severity. This system is used for classifying but not necessarily guiding therapy. Nonoperative management is successful in 94% of cases if the patient is hemodynamically stable.[20,40,41] Operative versus nonoperative management should be based on the clinical situation. Delayed bleeding can occur but is rare, reported in fewer than 2% of cases.[42]

*Return to play*

- Varies based on the grade of injury, with the higher-grade injuries taking longer to recover. Most experts recommend avoiding contact for 3 to 6 months. Liver studies should be back to normal. Follow-up CT scan can be considered to follow healing; however, is no longer routinely recommended unless clinically indicated.[20,38,43–45]

## Spleen

### Etiology and incidence

- The spleen is the most frequently injured organ, with blunt abdominal trauma in sports. The spleen lies behind the ninth to eleventh ribs in the left upper abdomen. In adults, the ribs provide some coverage, but in children, the spleen is not completely covered, putting kids at higher risk for injury.[46] Splenomegaly is common in athletes with mononucleosis. Spontaneous and traumatic rupture have been reported in up to 0.5% of cases with most occurring in the first 3 weeks from onset of symptoms.[47]

### Clinical examination

- Patients will typically present with left upper quadrant abdominal tenderness with rebound and guarding. The patient may complain of left shoulder pain ("Kehr sign"). Tachycardia and hypotension are late findings.

### Workup

- Serial abdominal examinations are important, as symptoms early on may be mild. FAST ultrasound examinations can be useful in detecting a hemoperitoneum. A CT scan is the imaging study of choice and can be used to grade injuries 1 to 5 based on severity.

### Treatment

- Patients should be admitted for observation with length of stay typically 1 day longer than the grade of injury.[46] The decision for surgical intervention is based on hemodynamic stability and should be considered in the more severe grade 4 and 5 injuries. Nonoperative treatment is more successful in children than in adults.[48] Risk of delayed rupture due to hemorrhage or pseudoaneurysm can occur in up to 8% of cases and up to 5 years out.[49,50] Patients with splenectomy may have a quicker return to sport.[51] Patients who undergo splenectomy must receive vaccination for encapsulated organisms including *Haemophilus influenza*, *Neisseria*, and *Pneumococcus*.

### Return to play

- Healing rate varies based on grade of injury, with higher-grade injuries taking longer. Light exercise may be initiated during the first 3 months. Contact sports should be avoided for 3 to 4 months, on average. CT scan and ultrasound can be used to follow healing rates, although are not routinely recommended.[52–55]

## Kidney

### Etiology and incidence

- Kidneys are the second-most commonly injured abdominal organ in sports. Most injures are due to direct blunt trauma to the back or flank and may be associated with rib and or spinous process fractures

### Clinical examination

- Patients may complain of back or flank pain and oftentimes have bruising overlying the injured area. Gross hematuria is suggestive, and 98% of injuries will have hematuria detected on urinalysis.[56,57]

### Workup

- A urinalysis should be obtained early in the workup and the presence of hematuria should prompt further imaging. FAST ultrasound examination may suggest hemoperitoneum, but CT scan imaging remains the study of choice. Similar to liver and spleen injuries, kidney injuries are graded 1 to 5 based on severity.

### Treatment

- All grade 1 and 2 injuries are managed nonoperatively with supportive management. Most grade 3 and 4 injuries can be managed without surgery as well. Grade 5 injuries are managed operatively.[58]

### Return to play

- Most injuries will heal within 6 to 8 weeks. Athletes should be withheld from sport until hematuria on urinalysis resolves, which varies from 2 to 4 weeks. Return to contact sports should be guided by urology consultation.[20,59] Athletes with a solitary kidney should be warned about risks of returning to contact and collision sports. Appropriate padding and protective wear should be encouraged.[60,61]

## Pancreas

### Etiology and incidence

- An insult to the pancreas is a rare injury accounting for fewer than 5% of all trauma cases and seldom recorded in sports literature, but is associated with high morbidity and mortality. The classic mechanism is compression of the pancreas against the spine due to blunt force.[62]

### Clinical examination

- Most patients present with abdominal pain, with only 10% having rebound pain.[62] Symptoms may be delayed as the pancreas sits retroperitoneal.

*Workup*

- CT scan imaging is the gold standard, although one study found a sensitivity of only 71% at detecting injury on initial scans.[63] In patients with persistent abdominal pain, consider repeat amylase and lipase laboratory tests, which are elevated on serial examinations in 89% of patients and potentially repeat CT scans if pain does not improve.[63]

*Treatment*

- Varies from conservative to surgical management based on CT findings and clinical symptoms.

*Return to play*

- Guarded. Guidelines not reported in the literature.[64]

### Bowel Injuries

*Etiology and incidence*

- Bowel injuries are rare in sports, compromising 1.1% of sports-related abdominal injuries. Small intestine injuries are more common than large intestine injuries. The mechanism can be from crush injury between the spine and a rigid object, or closed loop bursts, and shearing injuries from fixed positions.[65]

*Clinical examination*

- Initial examination may be benign, but a patient will continue to have persistent abdominal pain and eventually peritoneal signs. Fever, nausea, vomiting, tachycardia, rebound, and guarding also may be present.

*Workup*

- Patients may have an elevated white blood cell count. Early bowel injuries may be missed, but CT scan is the study of choice with the presence of free air and free fluid as early findings.[66]

*Treatment*

- Admission, antibiotics, and surgical management may be required. Delay in diagnosis may be associated with higher mortality and morbidity.

*Return to play*

- Varies based on individual cases, with most athletes able to return in 6 weeks.

### Scrotal/Testicular Injuries

*Etiology and incidence*

- Genitourinary injuries are rare, with nearly 75% of cases occurring in the pediatric patient population. Most injuries reported in a large cohort study involved a bicycle, but injuries are also common in football, baseball, hockey, and soccer. Sixty percent of injuries involve the external genitalia. Crush and direct blow injuries to the scrotum can cause testicular trauma, which should be rapidly assessed and diagnosed.[67]

*Clinical examination*

- Scrotal pain, swelling, and ecchymosis should prompt concern for underlying testicular rupture.

*Workup*

- Testicular ultrasound with Doppler is the study of choice to assess for underlying testicular rupture, testicular blood flow, and scrotal hematomas. These should be ordered emergently.

*Treatment*

- Testicular ruptures require surgery to increase the likelihood of preserving the testis. Early recognition, diagnostic ultrasound, and emergent surgical management/exploration are important for successful treatment.[68,69]

*Return to play*

- Athletes with a solitary testicle may return to sport but should be cautioned regarding future fertility and the use of cups/protective equipment should be strongly encouraged.

## REFERENCES

1. Reehal P. Facial injury in sport. Curr Sports Med Rep 2010;9(1):27–34.
2. Iida S, Kogo M, Sugiura T, et al. Retrospective analysis of 1502 patients with facial fractures. Int J Oral Maxillofac Surg 2001;30(4):286–90.
3. Neuman MI, Eriksson E. Facial trauma. In: Fleisher G, Henretig R, editors. Philadelphia: Lippincott Williams & Wilkins; 2005. p. 1475.
4. Büttner M, Schlittler FL, Michel C, et al. Is a black eye a useful sign of facial fractures in patients with minor head injuries? A retrospective analysis in a level I trauma centre over 10 years. Br J Oral Maxillofac Surg 2014;52(6):518–22.
5. Escott EJ, Branstetter BF. Incidence and characterization of unifocal mandible fractures on CT. AJNR Am J Neuroradiol 2008;29(5):890–4.
6. Neiner J, Free R, Caldito G, et al. Tongue blade bite test predicts mandible fractures. Craniomaxillofac Trauma Reconstr 2016;9(2):121–4.
7. Roccia F, Diaspro A, Nasi A, et al. Management of sport-related maxillofacial injuries. J Craniofac Surg 2008;19(2):377–82.
8. Basheeth N, Donnelly M, David S, et al. Acute nasal fracture management: a prospective study and literature review. Laryngoscope 2015;125(12):2677.
9. Esmaeli B, Elner SG, Schork MA, et al. Visual outcome and ocular survival after penetrating trauma. A clinicopathologic study. Ophthalmology 1995;102(3):393–400.
10. Zagelbaum BM, Starkey C, Hersh PS, et al. The National Basketball Association eye injury study. Arch Ophthalmol 1995;113:749–52.
11. Waldmen N, Densie IK, Herbison P, et al. Topical tetracaine used for 24 hours is safe and rated highly effective by patients for the treatment of pain caused by corneal abrasions: a double-blind, randomized clinical trial. Acad Emerg Med 2014;21(4):374–82.
12. Jacobsen B, Lahham S, Lahham S, et al. Retrospective review of ocular point-of-care ultrasound for detection of retinal detachment. West J Emerg Med 2016;17(2):196–200.
13. Glendor U. Epidemiology of traumatic dental injuries–a 12 year review of the literature. Dent Traumatol 2008;24(6):603–11.
14. Mueller FO, Cantu RC. Annual survey of catastrophic football injuries, 1977-2012. National Center for Catastrophic Sport Injury Research; 2012. Available at: http://nccsir.unc.edu/reports/.

15. Kepler CK, Vaccaro AR. Injuries and abnormalities of the cervical spine and return to play criteria. Clin Sports Med 2012;31(3):499–508.
16. Phillips NR, Kunz DE. Chest trauma in athletic medicine. Curr Sports Med Rep 2018;17:90–6.
17. Johnson BK, Comsock RD. Epidemiology of chest, rib thoracic spine, and abdomen injuries among United States high school athletes, 2005/2006 to 2013/2014. Clin J Sport Med 2017;27:388–93.
18. Chan SS. Emergency bedside ultrasound for the diagnosis of rib fractures. Am J Emerg Med 2009;27:617–20.
19. Turk F, Kurt AB, Saglam S. Evaluation by ultrasound of traumatic rib fractures missed by radiology. Emerg Radiol 2010;17:473–7.
20. Thomas RD, De Luigi AJ. Chest trauma in athletes. Curr Sports Med Rep 2018; 17(8):251–3.
21. Meese MA, Wayne JS. Pulmonary contusion secondary to blunt trauma in collegiate football player. Clin J Sport Med 1997;7:309–10.
22. Lively MW, Stone D. Pulmonary contusion in football players. Clin J Sport Med 2006;16:177–8.
23. Trupka A, Waydhas C, Hallfeldt KK, et al. Value of thoracic computed tomography in the first assessment of severely injured patients with blunt chest trauma: results of a prospective study. J Trauma 1997;43:405–11.
24. Feden JP. Closed lung trauma. Clin Sports Med 2013;32:255–65.
25. Partridge RA, Coley A, Boeie R, et al. Sports related pneumothorax. Ann Emerg Med 1997;30:539–41.
26. Inaba K, Branco BC, Eckstein M, et al. Optimal positioning for emergent needle thoracostomy: a cadaver-based study. J Trauma 2011;71(5):1099–103.
27. Sharma A, Jindal P. Principles of diagnosis and management of traumatic pneumothorax. J Emerg Trauma Shock 2008;1:34–41.
28. Kirkpatrick AW, Sirois M, Laupland KB, et al. Hand-held thoracic sonography for detecting post-traumatic pneumothoraces: the extended focused assessment with sonography for trauma (EFAST). J Trauma 2004;57:288–95.
29. Ianniello S, Di Giacoma V, Sessa B, et al. First line sonographic diagnosis of pneumothorax in major trauma: accuracy of e-FAST and comparison with multidetector computed tomography. Radiol Med 2014;119:674–80.
30. Chadha TS, Cohn MA. Non invasive treatment of pneumothorax with oxygen inhalation. Respiration 1983;44:147.
31. Aerospace Medical Associateion Medical Guidelines Task Force. Medical guidelines for airline travel, 2nd edition. Aviat Space Environ Med 2003;74(Suppl 5): A1–19.
32. Chaudhry S. Pediatric posterior sternoclavicular joint injuries. J Am Acad Orthop Surg 2015;23:468–75.
33. Bergqvist D, Hedelin H, Karlsson G, et al. Abdominal trauma during thirty years: analysis of a large case series. Injury 1981;13:93–9.
34. Thomson H, Francis DM. Abdominal wall tenderness: a useful sign in the acute abdomen. Lancet 1977;2:1053–4.
35. Johnson R. Abdominal wall injuries: rectus abdominis strains, oblique strains, rectus sheath hematoma. Curr Sports Med Rep 2006;5:99–103.
36. Amaral JF. Thoracoabdominal injuries in the athlete. Clin Sports Med 1997;16(4): 739–53.
37. Wan J, Corvind TF, Greenfield SP. Kidney and testicle injuries in team and individual sports: data from the national pediatric trauma registry. J Urol 2003;170: 1528–32.

38. Juyia RF, Kerr HA. Return to play after liver and spleen trauma. Sports Health 2014;6(3):239–45.
39. McKenney MG, Martin L, Lentz K, et al. 1000 consecutive ultrasounds for blunt abdominal trauma. J Trauma 1996;40(4):607–12.
40. Rifat SF, Gilfydis RP. Blunt abdominal trauma in sports. Curr Sports Med Rep 2003;2:93–7.
41. Pachter HL. The current status of nonoperative management of adult blunt hepatic injuries. Am J Surg 1995;169:442–54.
42. Parmelee-peters K, Moeller JL. Liver trauma in a high school football player. Curr Sports Med Rep 2004;3:95–9.
43. Karp MP. The nonoperative management of pediatric hepatic trauma. J Pediatr Surg 1983;18(4).
44. Tiberio GA. Evaluation of the healing time of non-operatively managed liver injuries. Hepatogastroenterology 2008;55:1010–2.
45. Ray R, Lemire J. Liver laceration in an intercollegiate football player. J Athl Train 1995;30:324–6.
46. Gaines BA. Intra-abdominal solid organ injury in children: diagnosis and treatment. J Trauma 2009;67:135–8.
47. Kindernecht JJ. Infectious mononucleosis and the spleen. Curr Sports Med Rep 2002;1:116–20.
48. Gannon EH, Howard T. Splenic injuries in athletes: a review. Curr Sports Med Rep 2010;9:111–4.
49. Clark OH, Lim RC. Spontaneous delayed splenic rupture—case report of a five year interval beween trauma and diagnosis. J Trauma 1975;15:245–9.
50. Frumiento C. Complications of splenic injuries: expansion of the nonoperative theorem. J Pediatr Surg 2000;35:788–91.
51. Terrell TR, Lundquist B. Management of splenic rupture and return to play decisions in a college football player. Clin J Sport Med 2002;12:400–42.
52. Pearl RH. Splenic injury: a 5 year update with improved results and changing criteria for conservative management. J Pediatr Surg 1989;24:428–31.
53. Savage SA. The evolution of blunt splenic injury: resolution and progression. J Trauma 2008;64:1085–92.
54. Pranikoff T, Hirschl RB. Resolution of splenic injury after nonoperative management. J Pediatr Surg 1994;29:1366–9.
55. Lynch JM, Meza MP, Newman B, et al. Computed tomography grade of splenic injury is predictive of the time required for radiographic healing. J Pediatr Surg 1997;32:1093–5.
56. Diamond DL. Sports related abdominal trauma. Clin J Sport Med 1989;8:91–9.
57. Miller KS, McAninch JW. Radiographic assessment of renal trauma: our 15 year experience. J Urol 1995;154:352–5.
58. Bernard JJ. Renal trauma: evaluation, management, and return to play. Curr Sports Med Rep 2009;8(2):98–103.
59. McAleer MJ. Renal and testis injuries in team sports. J Urol 2002;168:1805–7.
60. Papagiannopoulos D, Gong E. Revisiting sports precautions in children with solitary kidneys and congenital anomalies of the kidney and urinary tract. Urology 2016;101:9–14.
61. Zaydfudim V, Cotton BA, Kim BD. Pancreatic transection after sports injury. J Trauma 2010;69(4):33.
62. Bradley EL, Young PR, Chang MC, et al. Diagnosis and initial management of blunt pancreatic trauma. Guidelines from a multi-institutional review. Ann Surg 1998;227(6):861–9.

63. Echlin PS, Klein WB. Pancreatic injury in the athlete. Curr Sports Med Rep 2005;4: 96–101.
64. Williams MD, Watts D. Colon injury after blunt abdominal trauma: results of the EAST Multi-institutional hollow viscus injury study. J Trauma 2003;55:906–12.
65. Hughes TM, Elton C. The pathophysiology and management of bowel and mesenteric injuries due to blunt trauma. Injury 2002;33:295–302.
66. Bagga HS, fisher PB, Tasian GE, et al. Sports-related genitourinary injuries presenting to United States emergency departments. Urology 2015;85:239–44.
67. Fahlbusch B, Fahlbusch M, Thon WF. Blunt testicular injury—conservative or surgical treatment? Aktuell Urol 2003;34(3):176–8.
68. Wang Z, Yang JR, Huang YM, et al. Diagnosis and management of testicular rupture after blunt scrotal trauma: a literature review. Int Urol Nephrol 2016;48: 1967–76.
69. Freehill MT, Gorbachinsky I, Lavender JD, et al. Presumed testicular rupture during a college baseball game. Sports Health 2015;7(2):177–80.

# Supporting Mental Health and Well-being Among Student-Athletes

Karen P. Egan, PhD

## KEYWORDS

- Student-athlete mental health • Student-athlete well-being • Holistic care
- Integrative care

## KEY POINTS

- Although athletics participation provides multiple benefits that can be protective factors for mental health, stressors unique to athletics participation are also present.
- This article reviews the frequency and symptoms of the most common mental health concerns impacting collegiate student-athletes and discusses treatment approaches.
- This article reviews the importance of prioritizing mental health and well-being by trying to reduce stigma and provide access to qualified licensed providers.
- The value of multidisciplinary treatment teams and the ensuing coordination of care is also discussed.

## INTRODUCTION

Mental health and well-being is essential to being able to perform one's best within career, academics, relationships, and sport. Athletics provides multiple benefits that can be protective factors for mental health. Exercise has been found to reduce symptoms of anxiety and depression.[1,2] For collegiate student-athletes (SAs), starting fresh in the new college environment with a group of people they can get to know and spend time with for social support can help to ease the transition into college life and improve well-being. In addition, collegiate SAs frequently have access to a greater number of resources than their nonathlete peers by nature of their sport. For example, SAs may find support from coaches, teammates, and support staff, including physicians, certified athletic trainers, mental health providers, sports nutrition staff, operations staff, administrators, academic staff, and professors. Finally, working toward a goal or purpose through sport often adds meaning and value to many people's daily life. Conquering small goals each day can help individuals to see measurable progress for the work they put in and can serve to enhance self-esteem.

Disclosure Statement: The author has nothing to disclose.
University of Virginia Athletics Department, McCue Center, PO Box 400845, 290 Massie Road, Charlottesville, VA 22904-4845, USA
*E-mail address:* kpe4q@virginia.edu

Clin Sports Med 38 (2019) 537–544
https://doi.org/10.1016/j.csm.2019.05.003
0278-5919/19/© 2019 Elsevier Inc. All rights reserved.

However, a sport experience can also include a number of widespread stressors. Athletes experience the same stressors as their nonathlete peers, such as coping with symptoms of anxiety, mood disorders, challenges with eating behavior or substance use, gender-based violence or sexual assault, racism, and harassment or violence based on sexual orientation. Yet, in addition to these difficulties, athletes are often highly visible to others, particularly through social media, placing them in a more vulnerable position, and they may experience bullying, hazing, threats, harassment, and/or criticism because of this increased attention. This visibility can also impact body image and eating behavior in unique ways within the sport environment. Furthermore, for athletes there is often not only the expectation to perform at a high level, but also to win, a pressure that can come from within the athletes themselves, as well as from coaches, administrators, fans, or family members. Transitioning to the next level in sport (whether collegiate or professional) can also bring a reduced role on the team and reduced playing time. This position can create stress and a negative view of oneself if the athlete's previous identity was defined by success in sport. Athletic injury can also generate added stress because it often results in a mix of emotions typically highlighted by worry about returning to pre-injury level of competition,[3] isolation from teammates for a period of time,[4] and/or sadness or depressive symptoms.[5] Ironically, the same support systems that can be protective for athletes can also become a source of stress when conflict emerges with coaches and/or teammates. Transitioning out of sport owing to injury or illness or the end of one's playing career can also be a challenging adjustment. Exploring career options outside of athletics can prove challenging for SAs who have busy schedules and who may fear that coaches will view them as less committed if they explore career options outside of professional sport.

Depending on the level of sport being played, additional challenges may also be present. For collegiate SAs, the time demands of balancing the equivalent of 2 full-time jobs—academics and athletics—is a huge source of stress because the long hours decrease time for sleep and self-care. Travel time results in missed classes that have to be made up, and SAs often cannot access many resources available to nonathlete students during business hours owing to their schedules. Time demands among this population may also be increasing as a National Collegiate Athletic Association (NCAA) study found that collegiate SAs reported an increase in the time spent on both athletics and academics in 2015 as compared with 2010.[6] These division I SAs reported spending a median of 34 hours per week in season on athletics in 2015 versus 32 hours per week in season in 2010 while reporting a median of 38.5 hours per week on academics in-season in 2015 versus 35.5 hours per week in 2010.[6]

There exist differing stressors on other levels of sport participation. For middle and high school SA, for example, the burden of seeking collegiate scholarship opportunities can affect the younger athletes hoping to pursue their sporting and academic careers. On the other end of the spectrum, professional athletes may struggle with the time spent away from family, friends, and support systems owing to travel demands. These factors, in conjunction with the physical demands of sport, can prove to be exceedingly challenging.

Athletes often excel at embracing challenges, setting goals, making sacrifices to achieve these goals, staying motivated, and being open to feedback to help them improve. However, these same strengths can make some athletes reluctant to seek care owing to fear of negative perceptions. The stigma persists that mental health should be something that SAs can "push through" and "fix on their own" or that seeking care is a "sign of weakness," particularly among male SAs. Changing this stigma is essential to promoting the proactive use of mental health resources and prioritizing well-being.

## COMMON MENTAL HEALTH CONCERNS

Anxiety and depression are the most common mental health diagnoses among college students.[7] In a 2018 survey of college students with 88,178 respondents, 22.1% of respondents reported having been diagnosed or treated by a professional for anxiety and 18.1% diagnosed or treated by a professional for depression.[7] In this section, I focus on the most common mental health concerns impacting collegiate SAs, though many other symptoms can be present in SA populations as well. Symptoms can create a large disruption to well-being and functioning in relationships, academics, and athletics so identification and management are imperative for health.

### Anxiety Disorders

Approximately 87% of college student respondents to a 2018 survey said that they have "felt overwhelmed by all you had to do" and approximately 63% said that they have "felt overwhelming anxiety" at any time over the past 12 months.[7] When comparing collegiate SAs with nonathletes across 8 surveys from 2008 to 2012, fewer SAs reported experiencing anxiety than their nonathletes peers within the last 12 months (31% of male SAs vs 40% of male nonathletes and 48% of female SAs vs 56% of female nonathletes).[8] Although fewer SAs reported experiencing anxiety, nearly one-third of male SAs and nearly one-half of female SAs reported being impacted by anxiety, indicating this experience remains common among SAs.[8] Symptoms can range from mild to severe and may include feeling agitated, difficulty concentrating, irritability, physical distress, disruptions in sleep and/or appetite, panic attacks, phobias, obsessive thinking, and behavioral routines.[9] Anxiety symptoms can be connected to a specific topic, such as athletic performance, academic performance, or social interactions, but most commonly is experienced across multiple areas. SAs often defer self-care to prioritize athletic and academic obligations, which may enhance stress and worry because they frequently sacrifice much-needed time to decompress.

### Depressive Disorders

In the general population, roughly 7% of people are estimated to have experienced a major depressive disorder within the past 12 months with certain subpopulations having a greater incidence, namely, those between the ages of 18 and 29 experience major depressive disorder at a higher rate than older individuals and women experience major depressive disorder more often than men.[9] Looking more closely across the university setting, it is apparent that college students also struggle with depression. Approximately 53% of college students have reported they "felt things were hopeless," 63% "felt very lonely," 69% "felt very sad," and 42% "felt so depressed it was difficult to function" at any time over the past 12 months.[7] When comparing collegiate SAs with nonathletes across 8 surveys from 2008 to 2012, fewer SAs reported that they "felt depressed" than nonathletes within the last 12 months (21% of male SAs vs 27% of male nonathletes and 28% of female SAs vs 33% of female nonathletes).[8] Again, SAs reported fewer of these symptoms than their nonathlete peers; however, a significant portion of SAs did report having been impacted by depressive symptoms. Symptoms range in severity and may include feeling down, anhedonia, decreased motivation, fatigue, difficulty concentrating, disruptions in sleep and/or appetite, feelings of worthlessness, and/or suicidal ideation.[9] Depressive symptoms can make it feel nearly impossible to get out of bed each day and complete tasks, which can be particularly challenging for SAs who typically have many mandatory tasks each day.

Suicidal ideation can also occur with depressive symptoms or with other mental health concerns. At any time over the past 12 months, 12.1% of college student respondents endorsed that they have "seriously considered suicide," 1.7% "attempted suicide," and 7.8% "intentionally cut, burned, bruised, or otherwise injured" themselves.[7] Ensuring athletics staff and other SAs feel comfortable asking individuals directly about potential thoughts of suicide or self-harm and how to refer them to licensed mental health providers can help connect individuals to treatment providers quickly.

### Bipolar Disorders

Approximately 2% of college student survey respondents reported having been diagnosed or treated by a professional for bipolar disorder within the past 12 months.[7] Bipolar I disorder is defined as experiencing a manic episode has occurred, whereas bipolar II disorder is the presence of a hypomanic episode as well as a major depressive episode.[9] Hypomania is a symptom that can be overlooked at times, particularly in college environments where a decreased need for sleep and increase in goal-directed activity can be perceived as beneficial for short-term gains in academics or athletics. Recognizing symptoms early can help to decrease long-term risk and assist the SA to engage in treatment to promote their health and well-being.

### Substance Use

Approximately 1% of college student survey respondents reported having been diagnosed or treated by a professional for substance abuse or addiction to substances within the past 12 months.[7] NCAA studies have found that reported incidents of binge drinking among SAs have decreased over time (**Table 1**).

The highest rates of binge drinking were reported in lacrosse (69% of men, 57% of women), hockey (64% of men, 56% of women), and swimming (55% of men, 49% of women).[10] Marijuana use was reported to be the next most commonly used substance among SAs; 24% reported inhaling marijuana in the last year and 11% using edible forms.[10] For nicotine use in the past year, 17% of SAs reported smoking a cigar at least once, 13% used spit tobacco, 11% smoked cigarettes, 10% used hookah, and 8% used e-cigarettes.[10] Tobacco use was highest among male ice hockey and baseball players, with nearly 20% of male SAs in these sports reporting daily use.[10] These data came from 2017 and recent trends in the use of e-cigarettes may impact these data in the future. Substance abuse can result in an inability to complete academic and athletic obligations, harm relationships, and negatively impact mood, physical health, and financial health.

### Eating Behavior and Body Image

Concerning eating behaviors typically include restricting food intake, self-induced vomiting or other compensatory behaviors and/or binge eating. Among college students, 1.6% reported having been diagnosed or treated by a professional for anorexia nervosa and 1.2% for bulimia nervosa in the past 12 months.[7] Many SAs experience challenges in eating behavior and body image and can experience subclinical disturbances in eating behavior (often called disordered eating behavior) or can meet the

| Table 1 NCAA studies on drinking | | | |
|---|---|---|---|
| NCAA Research findings[10] | 2009 | 2013 | 2017 |
| Percentage of SAs who reported "binge drinking" (defined as ≥4 drinks in 1 sitting for women, ≥5 drinks in 1 sitting for men) | 55 | 51 | 42 |
| Percentage of SAs who reported drinking ≥10 drinks in 1 sitting | 15 | 12 | 8 |

diagnostic criteria for an eating disorder. Sometimes disturbances in eating behavior are difficult to detect among SAs where a focus on healthy eating and exercising above and beyond regular training is typically celebrated as progress toward athletic goals and good work ethic. Although eating disorders and disordered eating behavior occur across all sports, sports that have an increased risk fall into 2 categories: those that are judged in part on aesthetics where body size and shape can influence a score or evaluation (ie, gymnastics, diving, dance, cheer) and those that believe a lower weight will increase athletic performance (ie, distance running, distance swimming, rowing).[11] Another risk factor for athletes is revealing uniforms.[11] The added pressure of appearing in a small amount of clothing for competition, practice, and in media coverage of sport can be difficult to cope with. In addition, SAs may experience challenges when the media portrays a societal ideal body image that contradicts the ideal body image presented for their sport. This often impacts women in sports who require a higher body weight or greater muscularity and men in sports requiring a lower body weight or less muscularity. Negative body image is correlated with low self-esteem, depression, and the development of eating disorders and disordered eating behavior.[11]

### Gender-Based Violence and Sexual Assault

Gender-based violence, sexual assault, and other traumatic experiences also have a large impact on well-being and mental health. Symptoms may include flashbacks, nightmares, avoidance of reminders of the event, changes in mood, persistent negative cognitions, difficulty concentrating, sleep problems, reckless behavior, hypervigilance, and more.[9] Trauma experienced by an SA from a perpetrator who is also an SA or who is a staff member within the athletics department can have a particularly difficult impact on SAs' well-being. Additional experiences of trauma among peers, family members, and/or from others receiving coverage from news media can also trigger past experiences of trauma and result in current symptoms.

### Other

SAs are also impacted by psychosis, sleep disorders, personality disorders, attention-deficit hyperactivity disorder (see Mario Ciocca's article, "Attention Deficit Hyperactivity Disorder and Treatment for Athletes", in this issue for more information), and many other mental health concerns that impact the general population as well.

## TREATMENT

There are many well-established forms of psychotherapy from a number of different theoretic backgrounds that are effective for symptom reduction, improvement in quality of life, and improved relationships. Many forms of psychotherapy can be effective for working with SAs, such as cognitive-behavioral therapy, acceptance and commitment therapy, interpersonal therapy, positive psychology, humanistic therapy, and more. Although each approach differs in terms of how symptoms are conceptualized and the work is structured in therapy sessions, each approach can integrate aspects of athletic culture to adapt to each SA's needs. For example, cognitive-behavioral therapy may include helping SAs to identify their automatic negative thoughts and teaching them ways to use thought-challenging techniques to identify an alternative consideration that can then result in a change in their emotions and behaviors that impact mood, athletic performance, relationships, and academic performance.[12] As another example, positive psychology may focus on identifying an SA's strengths and capitalizing on those to make changes in thoughts, behaviors, and purpose as well. SAs often spend a lot of time and energy focusing on their weaknesses to identify areas to improve in athletics, so shifting their focus to increasing awareness of positive qualities they posses can provide them new tools to cope in moments of distress. Licensed mental health providers working with SAs ideally have experience working with individuals with a strong athletic identity[13] and should also be familiar with athletics culture to provide the best care.

To provide holistic care for SAs experiencing mental health concerns, collaboration between a multidisciplinary team of a licensed mental health provider, team physicians, certified athletic trainers, psychiatrists, and/or dieticians helps to ensures that everyone is working toward the same goals. For SAs taking psychiatric medications, coordination between the medical provider prescribing medication and the mental health provider doing psychotherapy with the client is particularly important for the health and well-being of the client. Collaboration is also essential for determining when participation in athletics should be limited for a period of time owing to mental health concerns. This limitation may be due to safety concerns and/or due to the severity of symptoms. Limited participation may be short term to allow an SA to reduce athletic stress while also prioritizing seeking mental health services. Participation may be limited for a longer period if an SA requires a higher level of care, such as an intensive outpatient program, partial hospitalization program, or inpatient services. Engaging supportive family members proves helpful as well. Many SAs communicate with parents frequently; 55% of collegiate SAs reported that they communicate with their parents once or more per day.[14] When SAs wish to sign a release of information document to coordinate care with specific family members, this can be another source of support for the SA. SAs may also request a mental health provider coordinate care with professors, academic coordinators, coaches, administrators, or other important individuals in their lives.

The early identification of SAs who could potentially benefit from psychotherapy can also help to get them connected to resources. Doing a preparticipation screening when SAs arrive on campus can allow SAs to self-identify that they wish to be connected to a licensed mental health provider and potentially identify SAs who may be struggling with mental health concerns.[15] Owing to the self-report nature of these screenings, these methods will inevitably not capture SAs who wish to hide potential symptoms owing to stigma and/or concern about their role in athletics or scholarship status.

## PROMOTING MENTAL HEALTH AND WELL-BEING

It is essential for SA well-being that mental health be prioritized at every level within the university and athletics department by working to reduce the stigma surrounding mental health concerns and by providing qualified resources accessible to all SAs. Stigma reduction is a key role for every medical provider, administrator, coach, staff member, and SA. Advocating for others to view seeking treatment as a sign of strength by acknowledging the courage it takes to be vulnerable helps to support SAs proactively seeking treatment. Every staff member and SA leader can address the importance of promoting mental health and well-being by partnering with mental health providers to:

- Normalize not feeling your best at all times.
- Provide educational material to teams.
- Share stories from other SAs and professional athletes who have chosen to speak publicly about their experiences with mental health concerns.
- Model the importance of self-care.

- Encourage SAs to engage in important conversations about mental health and how mental health is portrayed in sport culture and US culture.

Changing stigmatizing language within departments and teams can additionally have a large impact on well-being.

It is valuable for all staff members and SAs to be familiar with available licensed mental health providers and to know how to refer directly to these providers to encourage the use of these services. The NCAA Mental Health Best Practice Guidelines emphasizes the importance of planning in advance what procedures will exist for referring SAs to qualified licensed mental health providers.[15] Inviting licensed mental health providers to attend athletic events or give talks to athletic teams also helps to increase visibility to SAs and decrease potential barriers to seeking care. Those licensed mental health providers experienced in sport performance can additionally offer these skills to teams, which may also create more comfort for the SA reaching out to that provider for personal concerns as well. Some topics for performance work may include precompetition anxiety; coping with negative thoughts during practices, competition, or conditioning sessions; recovering from athletic injury; the use of visualization strategies; the use of mindfulness strategies; and sleep hygiene. SAs and staff members should also be familiar with how to contact licensed mental health providers in emergency situations.

Supporting mental well-being among SAs further involves observing SAs for signs of concern and then engaging them in a conversation about how they are doing. Potential signs of distress may include:

- Withdrawal from friends or activities
- Agitation or difficulty appearing calm
- Seeming to be down, sad, or having low energy
- Significant changes in eating behavior, sleep, and/or substance use
- Substantial weight loss or weight gain
- Making critical statements about oneself, one's value, and/or one's body shape, size, or weight
- Expressions of hopelessness
- Violent behavior
- Changes in personal hygiene
- Other statements of concern

Ideally someone who has a connection to the SA will approach them in a private setting or near-private setting. Private settings should not occur if the safety of the individual speaking to the SA would be comprised to meet one on one. A licensed mental health provider can train staff members and/or SA leaders about how to talk to an SA they are concerned about. A licensed mental health provider can teach communication strategies for this conversation, such as stating observed behaviors of concern, expressing care for the SA's well-being, using destigmatizing language, how to make a referral to a licensed mental health provider or medical provider with a background in mental health, assessing potential barriers to seeking care, discussing a plan to follow-up with the SA, and then following up afterward to see if they were able to get connected to a mental health provider.

Promoting a positive environment for mental health and well-being among SAs is an important mission for every athletics department to allow SAs to perform at their best socially, academically, and athletically. Every staff member and SA can actively take steps to decrease stigma and encourage discussions about mental health and well-being. Ensuring that all SAs can access care with a licensed mental health provider who understands the culture of sport and the importance of athletics in many SAs' identities can help ensure high quality care. Coordination of care among a multidisciplinary treatment team allows holistic care to ensure that SAs are able to focus on their personal and professional development goals.

## REFERENCES

1. Herring MP, Monroe DC, Fordon BR, et al. Acute exercise effects among young adults with analog generalized anxiety disorder. Med Sci Sports Exerc 2019. https://doi.org/10.1249/MSS.0000000000001860.
2. McCann IL, Holmes DS. Influence of aerobic exercise on depression. J Pers Soc Psychol 1984;46(5):1142–7.
3. Crossman J. Psychological rehabilitation from sports injuries. Sports Med 1997; 23(5):333–9.
4. Podlog L, Eklund RC. Professional coaches' perspectives on the return to sport following serious injury. J Appl Sport Psychol 2007;19:207–25.
5. Daly JM, Brewer BW, Van Raalte JL, et al. Cognitive appraisal, emotional adjustment, and adherence to rehabilitation following knee surgery. J Sport Rehabil 1995;4:23–30.
6. NCAA GOALS study of the student-athlete experience initial summary of findings. Available at: https://www.ncaa.org/sites/default/files/GOALS_2015_summary_jan 2016_final_20160627.pdf. Accessed November 21, 2018.
7. American College Health Association National College Health Assessment. Reference group executive summary 2018. Available at: https://www.acha.org/documents/ncha/NCHA-II_Spring_2018_Reference_Group_Executive_Summary. pdf. Accessed November 21, 2018.
8. NCAA. Mind, body, and sport: understanding and supporting student-athlete mental wellness. Available at: http://www.ncaapublications.com/p-4375-mind-body-and-sport-understanding-and-supporting-student-athlete-mental-wellness. aspx. Accessed November 21, 2018.
9. American Psychiatric Association. Diagnostic and statistical manual of mental disorders. 5th edition. Arlington (VA): American Psychiatric Association; 2013.
10. NCAA National Study on Substance Use Habits of College Student-Athletes. Executive summary June 2018. Available at: http://www.ncaa.org/sites/default/files/2017RES_Substance_Use_Executive_Summary_FINAL_20180611.pdf. Accessed November 21, 2018.
11. Thompson R, Sherman R. Eating disorders in sport. New York: Routledge Taylor & Frances Group; 2010.
12. Dobson KS, Dozois DJA. Historical and philosophical bases of the cognitive-behavioral therapies. In: Dobson KS, editor. Handbook of cognitive-behavioral therapies third edition (3-38). New York: The Guilford Press; 2010. p. 226–316.
13. Brewer BW, Van Raalte JL, Linder DE. Athletic identity: Hercules' muscles or Achilles heel? Int J Sport Psychol 1993;24:237–54.
14. NCAA Study of Student-Athlete Social Environments (2012-2016): January 2017 Preliminary Report. Available at: https://www.ncaa.org/sites/default/files/2017RES_NCAA_Convention_Social_Environments_present_20170807.pdf. Accessed November 21, 2018.
15. Interassociation consensus document: mental health best practices understanding and supporting student-athlete mental wellness. Available at: http://www.ncaa.org/sites/default/files/SSI_MentalHealthBestPractices_Web_20170921.pdf. Accessed December 10, 2018.

# Attention Deficit Hyperactivity Disorder in Athletes

Mario Ciocca, MD

## KEYWORDS

- Attention-deficit/hyperactivity disorder • Athletes • Stimulant medication
- Side effects • Banned medication

## KEY POINTS

- Attention-deficit/hyperactivity disorder (ADHD) can cause significant dysfunction academically, socially, and athletically if not properly treated.
- Stimulant medications are the first-line treatment of ADHD, although caution should be taken in prescribing because of the potential for side effects and misuse or abuse, which may affect athletic performance or could be life threatening.
- Treatment of ADHD can greatly benefit athletes, but physicians need to ensure a proper and comprehensive work-up is completed because there is no standard objective measure to diagnose ADHD and there is a high rate of comorbidity.
- It is important for physicians to properly educate athletes on the use and side effects of medications and to monitor these athletes through treatment.

## ATTENTION-DEFICIT/HYPERACTIVITY DISORDER

Attention-deficit/hyperactivity disorder (ADHD) is defined by certain attentional behaviors or symptoms in the Diagnostic and Statistical Manual of Mental Disorders (DSM). There are 3 categories: predominantly inattentive, showing at least 6 of the 9 inattention symptoms listed later; hyperactive/impulsive, showing at least 6 of the 9 hyperactive symptoms listed later; and combined type, showing symptoms of both inattention and hyperactivity.[1] Symptoms are present for a minimum of 6 months, initially developed before 12 years of age, and cause an effect across 2 or more settings.[1]

The 9 symptoms of inattention are:[1]

1. Failing to give close attention to details or making careless mistakes
2. Difficulty sustaining attention in tasks

Disclosure: The author has no relationship with a commercial company that has a direct financial interest in the subject matter or materials discussed in this article or with a company making a competing product.

Orthopeadics and Internal Medicine, UNC Sports Medicine, James A Taylor Campus Health Service, CB#7470, Chapel Hill, NC 27599, USA

E-mail address: ciocca@email.unc.edu

Clin Sports Med 38 (2019) 545–554
https://doi.org/10.1016/j.csm.2019.05.004
0278-5919/19/© 2019 Elsevier Inc. All rights reserved.

3. Often not listening when spoken to directly
4. Often not following through on instructions
5. Often having difficulties organizing tasks and activities
6. Often avoids or is reluctant to engage in tasks that require sustained mental effort
7. Often losing things that are necessary for tasks
8. Often easily distracted by extraneous stimuli
9. Often forgetful in daily activities

Symptoms of hyperactivity and impulsivity include:[1]

1. Often fidgets with hands/feet or squirms in seat
2. Often leaves seat when remaining in seat is expected
3. Often runs or climbs in situations in which it is inappropriate
4. Often unable to play or engage in leisure activities quietly
5. Often "on the go"
6. Often talks excessively
7. Often blurts out an answer before a question has been completed
8. Often has difficulty waiting to take a turn
9. Often interrupts or intrudes on others

## EPIDEMIOLOGY

Variations in prevalence exist across states, regions, and countries and are based on which criteria and assessments are used.[2] Prevalence rates vary between 1% and 10% in children and adolescents, with higher rates in boys and possibly athletes.[3,4] Fifty percent of children and adolescents continue to have symptoms as an adult.[5] A recent meta-analysis found a prevalence rate of 7.2%.[2] Over the last 25 years, the prevalence has increased, with more patients being diagnosed and treated.[6]

## ASSESSMENT

Variances in prevalence are partly caused by the lack of standard objective measures to diagnose ADHD. Assessment should include a history, physical, and standardized symptom questionnaires for not only the patient but also parents, teachers, or others involved in care.[7] The assessment should also evaluate for other conditions that may coexist, including mental health, learning or language disorders, and physical conditions.[7]

Individuals with untreated ADHD may have significant academic and social impairments. ADHD in children and adolescents is associated with reduced school performance and academic attainment, whereas in adults it is associated with poorer occupational performance and higher probability of unemployment.[1] Children and adolescents with ADHD are more likely to develop conduct disorder and antisocial personality, have a higher likelihood of substance use disorder, and have higher rates of incarceration.[1] With an increase in impulsivity and a decrease in focus, there is a higher likelihood of injury and an increased frequency of traffic violations and traffic accidents.[1]

## TREATMENT

Treatment of ADHD includes behavioral therapy to develop skills to reduce distractibility, cognitive behavior therapy, educational interventions, and education on the condition.[3,8] In addition, exercise alleviates symptoms of ADHD and the greatest effect is seen with mixed exercise programs.[9] With short-term exercise, there are improvements in response time, impulsivity, and attention. The long-term effects of exercise include a reduction in the severity of ADHD symptoms and a positive effect on executive function.[9,10]

The most common treatment of ADHD is psychotropic medication.[11] In children and adolescents, medications shown to be superior to placebo include amphetamines, atomoxetine, bupropion, clonidine, guanfacine, methylphenidate, and modafinil.[12] Medications that are effective in adults include amphetamine, methylphenidate, bupropion, and atomoxetine, whereas modafinil has not been superior to placebo.[12] When taking into account efficacy, safety, and tolerability, first-line medications include methylphenidate for children and amphetamines for adults.[12–14]

Stimulants act by blocking the transporter reuptake of both dopamine and norepinephrine.[15] Although stimulants may cause increased levels of dopamine in areas of the brain associated with drug abuse, when taken as prescribed the effect of stimulants mainly act in the prefrontal cortex.[15] This area controls arousal, attention, and inhibitory processes.[3] Therefore, treatment of ADHD reduces symptoms of hyperactivity, impulsivity, and inattention, and reduces executive dysfunction.[16] Effective treatment can improve quality of life, academic performance, rate of substance abuse, driving errors, and the prevalence of comorbid psychological disorders.[17]

## BENEFITS AND RISKS

Athletes with ADHD may benefit from treatment. The increase in focus and attention is beneficial for on-field tasks as well as off-field instruction and the ability to be coached. In addition, fine motor coordination and balance are improved.[3] Other general benefits of treatment include help with oppositional behavior, argumentative attitude, frustration, poor self-esteem, and mood lability.[18] Although the positive effects can be beneficial to athletes, there are potential side effects that may detract from performance and/or cause a risk to the health of the athlete. Stimulants can have an effect on sleep, cardiovascular system, gastrointestinal system, bone health, and thermoregulation. Additional caution regarding the use of stimulants includes the potential for misuse and abuse, including using medication for athletic enhancement.

## CARDIOVASCULAR

A primary concern with prescribing stimulants in athletes is the potential for serious cardiovascular effects. Stimulants can increase systolic blood pressure (3–5 mm Hg), diastolic blood pressure (2–14 mm Hg) and pulse (3–10 beats/min),[19] although there may be some differences between amphetamines and methylphenidate.[20] Although there have been case reports of sudden cardiac death related to ADHD medications, large cohort studies have not confirmed a link between stimulants and serious cardiovascular adverse events.[19] A more recent meta-analysis could not confirm a relationship between ADHD medications and stroke, myocardial infarction, or all-cause death but did show a positive association between ADHD medication and sudden death/arrhythmia.[21] The potential increase in blood pressure, heart rate, and chronic cardiovascular stress caused by stimulants, combined with the cardiovascular stress from intense exercise, should encourage physicians to appropriately screen for underlying cardiovascular disease. Athletes should be educated on risk and appropriate use and be monitored closely during treatment.

## SLEEP

Stimulants can cause sleep disruption, with increasing rates at progressively higher doses.[22] Proper sleep positively affects athletes in multiple ways ,whereas disruption of sleep can lead to a change in health and performance. Restriction, deprivation, or loss of sleep can have an effect on skill execution, submaximal strength, muscular and anaerobic power, time to exhaustion, alertness, reaction time, memory, and decision making.[23] Other negative effects of poor sleep include poorer overall mood and possible effects on illness and injury occurrence.[23] Caution needs to be taken on the time of day a stimulant is taken as well as its duration of action.

## BONE HEALTH

Another concern for athletes is the potential effect stimulant medication has on bone health. There is evidence that children and adolescents taking ADHD medications have a decrease in bone mineral density in the femoral neck, total femur, and lumbar spine compared with those not on stimulant medications.[24] The mechanism may include both direct agonist effects of the sympathetic nervous system and/or indirect effects on nutritional status.[24] Despite these changes in bone mineral density associated with stimulant medications, untreated ADHD is also associated with a higher risk of fracture. This higher risk arises because fracture risk is mitigated in those treated with ADHD medications by decreasing distractibility, decreasing substance abuse, improving frustration tolerance and self-esteem, and decreasing risk-taking behavior.[25] There is some evidence for an increase in stress fracture rates associated with stimulant medication use.[26]

## HEAT ILLNESS

A major concern with stimulant medication is the increased risk for heat illness. Athletes taking stimulant medication who exercise in high ambient temperature may modify the perception of effort and thermal stress, leading to an increase in core temperature.[27] Physicians need to properly educate athletes about this risk, particularly those who exercise at increased temperature and/or humidity and may have other risk factors, such as increased body mass, use of equipment restricting heat dissipation, or underlying medical problems.

## GASTROINTESTINAL

With regard to gastrointestinal tract function, bothersome side effects from stimulant therapy include nausea, abdominal pain, and anorexia,[28] which can lead to weight loss.[12] These side effects are a concern for athletes who either need to maintain weight for their sport or struggle to meet the caloric demands for exercise and performance.

## ABUSE AND MISUSE

Athletes with ADHD who are treated with stimulant medication benefit from the mitigation of symptoms but may seek a secondary gain to use stimulant medication as a performance enhancer outside of ADHD treatment. Amphetamines have been used by athletes to increase alertness, delay fatigue, and provide a feeling of aggressiveness.[29] Amphetamines may increase strength, muscle power, speed, acceleration, aerobic power, and anaerobic capacity, and improve reaction time when fatigued.[30,31] In addition, amphetamines can mask pain from injury, allowing athletes to continue competing and possibly exacerbating injuries.[31] Physicians need to remain alert for athletes seeking secondary gain and have an awareness of those trying to malinger and use an ADHD diagnosis to obtain stimulant medication. Periodic evaluation of the athlete should be completed and education given on proper use of stimulant medication.

Physicians need to be aware of diversion of medication and the nonmedical use of stimulants. Athletes may be on the receiving or giving end of medication sharing. Although stimulants may be misused for athletic performance, they may also be misused for academic performance in individuals who do not have an ADHD diagnosis. Stimulants may increase quality of note taking, scores on quizzes and worksheets, writing output, and homework completion.[5] Outside of performance, stimulants are misused recreationally and used as a party drug. In addition, misuse can be related to disordered eating. This possibility is of particular concern in athletes, especially those involved in sports in which either weight or body image may be stressed. Stimulant misuse has been associated with greater severity of global eating disorder, weight and body image concerns, binge eating and purging, eating disorder–related clinical impairment, depression, stress, and anxiety.[32]

In college students, the rate of misuse of prescription stimulants is around 17%.[33] This rate includes students that use medication without a prescription and those with a prescription who are using more than was prescribed. Among those that obtain stimulants for nonmedical use, most obtain it through sharing, but they may also obtain it through black market sources or misleading or manipulating a physician to write a prescription.[34] Those that do misuse and take higher doses than prescribed are at risk for psychosis, seizure, and cardiovascular events, including hypertension, tachycardia, cardiomyopathy, cardiac dysrhythmias, and necrotizing vasculitis.[5]

## NONSTIMULANT MEDICATION

Nonstimulant options for the treatment of ADHD include bupropion, clonidine, guanfacine, and atomoxetine.[11] Among physician members of the International Society for Sports Psychiatry, atomoxetine is the first-line choice for the treatment of ADHD in athletes, followed by long-acting stimulants.[35] This choice is influenced by concerns about performance enhancement, regulation by governing bodies, and safety.[35] Atomoxetine is a selective inhibitor of the norepinephrine transporter and increases the concentration of synaptic norepinephrine and dopamine in the prefrontal cortex.[36] Responses to atomoxetine tend to build over time and may not be maximal until after 3 months of treatment.[36] Given the mechanism of action, some of the side effects are similar to those of stimulants, including increases in systolic blood pressure, diastolic blood pressure, and heart rate; nausea; and decrease in appetite. Other side effects include dry mouth, fatigue, urinary hesitation, and erectile dysfunction.[37]

Clonidine has shown superiority compared with placebo for the treatment of ADHD.[38] Clonidine is a nonselective alpha-2 adrenergic agonist.[38] Alpha-2 adrenergic receptors are present in the prefrontal cortex, with the subtype alpha-2A mediating inattentiveness, hyperactivity, and impulsivity.[38] Clonidine can be used as monotherapy or as an adjunct to stimulants.[38] Side effects include dizziness, somnolence, bradycardia, and hypotension.[38]

Guanfacine works similarly to clonidine and is selective to the 2A receptor.[39] It also can be used as monotherapy or an adjunct to stimulant treatment and the side effects are similar to clonidine.[39] There is a high incidence of side effects causing noncompliance, and long-term efficacy and safety are unknown.[39] Another option is bupropion, which is used as an antidepressant. There is low-quality evidence that bupropion decreases the severity of ADHD symptoms and modestly increases the proportion of participants achieving a significant clinical improvement in ADHD symptoms.[40]

## CONCUSSION

Sports-related concussion is a traumatic brain injury induced by biomechanical forces.[41] Sport-related concussion typically results in the rapid onset of short-lived impairment in neurologic function that resolves spontaneously.[41] Concussions present with a variety of symptoms, many of which overlap with ADHD. This overlap may complicate the evaluation and assessment of athletes with ADHD who are concussed.

Athletes with ADHD have a higher prevalence of prior concussion than those without ADHD[42,43] and are more likely to report a history of greater than 3 concussions.[44] In those with ADHD, it is even more important to have a validated assessment tool for concussion given the increase in frequency and the overlap of symptoms with both of these conditions. Neuropsychological testing is frequently used as an assessment tool in athletes with concussion. Athletes with ADHD perform worse on baseline neurocognitive tests, including visual motor speed, visual memory, and reaction time, and report greater total symptom scores than those without ADHD.[45] Reported symptoms include difficulty concentrating, fatigue, trouble sleeping, difficulty remembering, balance problems, and the feeling of being in a fog.[44,46]

Following a concussion, athletes with ADHD have lower neuropsychological scores compared with athletes without ADHD.[45] In addition, those with ADHD have a higher symptom score and reported feeling more confused, feeling more slowed down, and having poorer concentration.[46] Note also that those with ADHD are more likely to produce an invalid protocol on neuropsychological testing.[47]

Medication can affect performance on neuropsychological testing. Athletes that are treated still perform worse on verbal memory and visual memory at baseline and after concussion[45] but do show improved measures on psychomotor speed and reaction time.[48]

Recovery from concussion usually occurs within a month after the injury.[41] A small minority of athletes report symptoms for multiple months after a concussion.[41] Multiple factors are associated with a prolonged recovery. ADHD has been discussed as a factor, although studies do not support this. Athletes with ADHD average 3 days longer in recovery time from concussion.[46] In addition, 1 study showed that a previous diagnosis of ADHD is associated with a higher risk of postconcussive symptoms lasting more than 28 days,[49] although multiple other studies have failed to show a substantially greater risk for persistent symptoms beyond 1 month.[50]

## ORGANIZATIONAL OVERSIGHT

Most governing bodies of sports organizations have regulations on the use of stimulant medication, and these are banned for in-competition use. Physicians should be familiar with the rules governing the relevant sport and take the precautions needed to adequately treat the athlete. Regulations are different for collegiate athletes under the National Collegiate Athletic Association (NCAA) compared with various professional organizations and compared with those under the International Olympic Committee and World Anti-Doping Agency (WADA). For those under the NCAA, stimulants are banned in competition, but athletes taking stimulants for ADHD can obtain a medical exception by using the NCAA medical exception documentation reporting form.[51] Preapproval is not necessary but a record needs to be kept on the diagnosis, course of treatment, and current prescription.[52] In addition, an appropriate comprehensive clinical evaluation needs to performed and documented, including individual and family history, assessment for comorbid conditions, previous history of ADHD treatment, using the DSM criteria to diagnose attention-deficit/hyperactivity disorder, and any supporting documentation such as ADHD rating scales.[52] If the athlete tests positive, then the documentation is sent to the NCAA.[51]

WADA also bans stimulant medications in competition.[53] A Therapeutic Use Exemption (TUE) needs to be filled out to obtain approval for use. A TUE is submitted to the antidoping organization and is then reviewed by a committee and either approved or denied.[54] Most organizations under WADA began granting TUEs for ADHD by 2008.[55] WADA recognizes the benefits of stimulant medications for ADHD and does not require a nonstimulant trial before using stimulants.[55] A TUE is usually granted for 1 year for athletes not on a stable dose of medication but may be granted for up to 4 years if on stable dosing.[55]

## SUMMARY

ADHD is just as prevalent in athletes as in the general population. Given the lack of objective measures for ADHD, assessment should be thorough and include corroboration from others and an assessment for comorbid conditions. Physicians should be aware of athletes who feign symptoms for personal gain. Although atomoxetine is a good alternative, the most effective treatment is stimulants. Physicians must be cautious and educate athletes on the potential side effects and proper use, warn about the diversion of medications, and be familiar with the banned substances for the governing body of the athlete's sport. When medications are used properly and with supervision, athletes with ADHD benefit socially, academically, and athletically.

## REFERENCES

1. American Psychiatric Association. The diagnostic and statistical manual of mental disorders. 5th edition. Washington, DC: American Psychiatric Association; 2013.
2. Thomas R, Sanders S, Doust J, et al. Prevalence of attention-deficit/hyperactivity disorder: a systematic review and meta-analysis. Pediatrics 2015;135(4): e994–1001.
3. Hickey G, Fricker P. Attention deficit hyperactivity disorder, CNS stimulants and sport. Sports Med 1999;27(1):11–21.
4. Nazeer A, Mansour M, Gross KA. ADHD and adolescent athletes. Front Public Health 2014;2(46):1–7.
5. Lakhan SE, Kirchgessner A. Prescription stimulants in individuals with and without attention deficit hyperactivity disorder: misuse, cognitive impact, and adverse effects. Brain Behav 2012;2(5):661–77.
6. Fairman KA, Peckham AM, Sclar DA. Diagnosis and treatment of ADHD in the United States: update by gender and race. J Atten Disord 2017. https://doi.org/10.1177/1087054716688534:1-10.
7. Wolraich M, Brown L, Brown RT, et al. ADHD: clinical practice guideline for the diagnosis, evaluation, and treatment of attention-deficit/hyperactivity disorder in children and adolescents. Pediatrics 2011;128(5):1007–22.
8. Kutcher JS. Treatment of attention-deficit hyperactivity disorder in athletes. Curr Sports Med Rep 2011;10(1):32–6.
9. Ng QX, Ho CYX, Chan HW, et al. Managing childhood and adolescent attention-deficit/hyperactivity disorder (ADHD) with exercise: a systematic review. Complement Ther Med 2017;34:123–8.

10. Hoza B, Martin CP, Pirog A, et al. Using physical activity to manage ADHD symptoms: the state of the evidence. Curr Psychiatry Rep 2016;18(12):113.

11. DuPaul GJ, Pollack B, Pinho TD. Attention-deficit/hyperactivity disorder. In: Goldstein S, Devries M, editors. Handbook of DSM-5 disorders in children and adolescents. Cham (Switzerland): Springer; 2017. p. 399–416.

12. Cortese S, Adamo N, Del Giovane C, et al. Comparative efficacy and tolerability of medications for attention-deficit hyperactivity disorder in children, adolescents, and adults: a systematic review and network meta-analysis. Lancet Psychiatry 2018;5:727–38.

13. Castells X, Blanco-Silvente L, Cunill R. Amphetamines for attention deficit hyperactivity disorder (ADHD) in adults (review). Cochrane Database Syst Rev 2018;(8):CD007813.

14. Punja S, Shamseert L, Hartling L, et al. Amphetamines for attention deficit hyperactivity disorder (ADHD) in children and adolescents (Review). Cochrane Database Syst Rev 2016;(2):CD009996.

15. Clemow DB, Walker DJ. The potential for misuse and abuse of medications in ADHD: a review. Postgrad Med 2014;126(5):64–81.

16. De Crescenzo F, Cortese S, Adamo N, et al. Pharmacological and non-pharmacological treatment of adults with ADHD: a meta-review. Evid Based Ment Health 2017;20(1):4–11.

17. Stewman CG, Liebman C, Fink L, et al. Attention deficit hyperactivity disorder: unique considerations in athletes. Sports Health 2018;10(1):40–6.

18. White RD, Harris GD, Gibson ME. Attention deficit hyperactivity disorder and athletes. Sports Health 2014;5(2):149–56.

19. Schneider BN, Enenbach M. Managing the risks of ADHD treatment. Curr Psychiatry Rep 2014;16(10):479.

20. Hennissen L, Bakker MJ, Banaschewski T, et al. Cardiovascular effects of stimulant and non-stimulant medication for children and adolescents with ADHD: a systematic review and meta-analysis of trials of methylphenidate, amphetamines and atomoxetine. CNS Drugs 2017;31:199–215.

21. Liu H, Feng W, Zhang D. Association of ADHD medications with the risk of cardiovascular disease: a meta-analysis. Eur Child Adolesc Psychiatry 2018. https://doi.org/10.1007/s00787-018-1217-x.

22. Becker SP, Froehlich TE, Epstein JN. Effects of methylphenidate on sleep functioning in children with attention-deficit/hyperactivity disorder. J Dev Behav Pediatr 2016;37(5):395–404.

23. Fullagar HHK, Skorski S, Duffield R, et al. Sleep and athletic performance: the effects of sleep loss on exercise performance, and psychological and cognitive response to exercise. Sports Med 2015;45:161–86.

24. Howard JT, Walick KS, Rivera JC. Preliminary evidence of an association between ADHD medications and diminished bone health in children and adolescents. J Pediatr Orthop 2017;37(5):348–54.

25. Perry BA, Archer KR, Song Y, et al. Medication therapy for attention deficit/hyperactivity disorder is associated with lower risk of fracture: a retrospective cohort study. Osteoporos Int 2016;27:2223–7.

26. Schermann H, Ben-Ami IS, Tudor A, et al. Past methylphenidate exposure and stress fractures in combat soldiers a case control study. Am J Sports Med 2018;46(3):728–33.

27. Roelands B, Hasegawa H, Watson P, et al. The effects of acute dopamine reuptake inhibition on performance. Med Sci Sports Exerc 2008;40(5):879–85.

28. Holmskov M, Storebo OJ, Moreira-Maia CR, et al. Gastrointestinal adverse events during methylphenidate treatment of children and adolescents with attention deficit hyperactivity disorder: a systematic review with meta-analysis and trial sequential analysis of randomised clinical trials. PLoS One 2017;12(6):e0178187.

29. Liddle DG, Connor DJ. Nutritional supplements and ergogenic AIDS. Prim Care 2013;40:487–505.

30. Chandler JV, Blair SN. The effect of amphetamines on selected physiological components related to athletic success. Med Sci Sports Exerc 1980;12:65–9.

31. Avois L, Robinson N, Saudan C, et al. Central nervous system stimulants and sport practice. Br J Sports Med 2006;40(suppl 1):16–20.

32. Gibbs EL, Kass AE, Eichen DM, et al. ADHD-specific stimulant misuse, mood, anxiety, and stress in college-age women at high risk for or with eating disorders. J Am Coll Health 2016;64(4):300–8.

33. Benson K, Flory K, Humphreys KL, et al. Misuse of stimulant medication among college students: a comprehensive review and meta-analysis. Clin Child Fam Psychol Rev 2015;18:50–76.

34. Vrecko S. Everyday drug diversions: a qualitative study of the illicit exchange and non-medical use of prescription stimulants on a university campus. Soc Sci Med 2015;131:297–304.

35. Reardon CL, Creado S. Psychiatric medication preferences of sports psychiatrists. Phys Sportsmed 2016;44(4):397–402.

36. Savill NC, Buitelaar JK, Anand E, et al. The efficacy of atomoxetine for the treatment of children and adolescents with attention-deficit/hyperactivity disorder: a comprehensive review of over a decade of clinical research. CNS Drugs 2015; 29:131–51.

37. Fredriksen M, Halmoy A, Faraone SV, et al. Long-term efficacy and safety of treatment with stimulants and atomoxetine in adult ADHD: a review of controlled and naturalistic studies. Eur Neuropsychopharmacol 2013;23:508–27.

38. Naguy A. Clonidine use in psychiatry: panacea or panache. Pharmacology 2016; 98(1–2):87–92.

39. Guanfacine for ADHD in children and adolescents. Drug Ther Bull 2016;5:56–60.

40. Verbeeck w, Bekkering GE, Van den Noortgate W, et al. Bupropion for attention deficit hyperactivity disorder (ADHD) in adults. Cochrane Database Syst Rev 2017;(10):CD009504.

41. McCrory P, Meeuwisse W, Dvorak J, et al. Consensus statement on concussion in sport-the 5th international conference on concussion in sport held in Berlin. 2016. Br J Sports Med 2018;51:838–47.

42. Iverson GL, Wojtowicz M, Brooks BL, et al. High school athletes with ADHD and learning difficulties have a greater lifetime concussion history. J Atten Disord 2016 [pii:1087054716657410].

43. Brett BL, Kuhn AW, Yengo-Kahn AM, et al. Risk factors associated with sustaining a sport-related concussion: an initial synthesis study of 12,320 student-athletes. Arch Clin Neuropsychol 2018;33:984–92.

44. Nelson LD, Guskiewicz KM, Marshall SW, et al. Multiple self-reported concussions are more prevalent in athletes with ADHD and learning disability. Clin J Sport Med 2016;26:120–7.

45. Gardner RM, Yengo-Kahn A, Bonfield CM, et al. Comparison of baseline and post-concussion ImPACT test scores in young athletes with stimulant-treated and untreated ADHD. Phys Sportsmed 2017;45:1–10.

46. Poysophon P, Rao AL. Neurocognitive deficits associated with ADHD in athletes: a systematic review. Sports Health 2018;10(4):317–26.

47. Manderino L, Gunstad J. Collegiate student athletes with history of ADHD or academic difficulties are more likely to produce an invalid protocol on baseline ImPACT testing. Clin J Sport Med 2018;28(2):111–6.
48. Littleton AC, Schmidt JD, Register-Mihalik JK, et al. Effects of attention deficit hyperactivity disorder and stimulant medication on concussion symptom reporting and computerized neurocognitive test performance. Arch Clin Neuropsychol 2015;30:683–93.
49. Miller JH, Gill CD, Kuhn EN, et al. Predictors of delayed recovery following pediatric sports related concussion: a case-control study. J Neurosurg Pediatr 2016; 17(4):491–6.
50. Iverson GL, Gardner AJ, Terry DP, et al. Predictors of clinical recovery from concussion: a systematic review. Br J Sports Med 2017;51:941–8.
51. NCAA sport science institute drug policies for your health and safety. Available at: http://www.ncaa.org/sites/default/files/SSI2018-19_Drug_Policies_Brochure_20180 706.PDF. Accessed December 5, 2018.
52. NCAA medical exception documentation reporting form to support the diagnosis of attention deficit hyperactivity disorder (ADHD) and treatment with banned stimulant medication. Available at: http://www.ncaa.org/sites/default/files/2018-19SSI_ADHA_Medical_Exceptions_Reporting_Form_20180710.pdf. Accessed December 5, 2018.
53. The world anti-doping code international standard prohibited list January 2019. Available at: https://www.wada-ama.org/sites/default/files/wada_2019_english_prohibited_list.pdf. Accessed December 5, 2018.
54. Frequently Asked Questions (FAQ). Therapeutic use exemptions (TUEs) November 17, 2016. Available at: https://www.wada-ama.org/sites/default/files/resources/files/2016-11-17-qa_tues_en_0.pdf. Accessed December 5, 2018.
55. White S. TUEs for ADHD WADA TUEC Chairs Symposium – Paris 2014. Available at: https://www.wada-ama.org/sites/default/files/resources/files/06-_white_susan_-_adhd_paris_symposium.pdf. Accessed December 5, 2018.

# Infectious Mononucleosis Management in Athletes

Anthony S. Ceraulo, DO[a,b,1], Jeffrey R. Bytomski, DO[a,b,*]

## KEYWORDS

- Infectious mononucleosis • Athlete • Return to play • Ultrasound

## KEY POINTS

- Infectious mononucleosis is a common problem encountered in the athletic training room, affecting a significant percentage of high school and collegiate athletes annually.
- The most effective way to manage infectious mononucleosis involves using common history and clinical indicators, screening tests, and diagnostic laboratories
- Return to play decisions with infectious mononucleosis are complicated by the small risk of splenic rupture, which may be best quantified with the use of serial ultrasonography

## INTRODUCTION

Infectious mononucleosis (IM) is a relatively common condition associated with athletic training rooms. Clinicians are often aware of the classic clinical findings and the need for recognition; however, much debate has existed over the years regarding safe return to play (RTP) guidelines.

## EPIDEMIOLOGY

IM is a condition associated with several different viral origins. The most commonly implicated is Epstein-Barr virus (EBV), which is a herpesvirus that is primarily transmitted via intimate person to person contact, which accounts for nearly 90% of cases of IM. EBV is present in the salivary glands for months after acute illness, leading to saliva as a common source of transmission. There has also been some evidence to suggest sexual transmission and breastfeeding as potential methods owing to isolation of the virus in the involved media. Exposure to EBV is almost uniform; some studies have suggested upward of 95% EBV antibody seropositivity by adulthood as a result of such high exposure rates. Many are exposed in their childhood years,

Disclosure: There are no financial or personal disclosures to report.
a Department of Community and Family and Medicine, Duke University, Durham, NC, USA;
b Department of Orthopedics, Duke University, Durham, NC, USA
1 Present address: 76 Intuition Circle, Durham, NC 27705.
* Corresponding author. Duke University Medical Center, Box 3672, Durham, NC 27708.
E-mail address: jeffrey.bytomski@duke.edu

Clin Sports Med 38 (2019) 555–561
https://doi.org/10.1016/j.csm.2019.06.002
0278-5919/19/© 2019 Elsevier Inc. All rights reserved.

sportsmed.theclinics.com

and often the infection is subclinical and therefore goes unnoticed. In symptomatic cases, once exposed, the viral incubation period is approximately 4 to 8 weeks until the onset of clinical symptoms in the exposed individual.

Of note, EBV-negative IM is associated with a variety of other infections. This article focusses primarily on EBV; however, it should be noted that primary infection with HIV, CMV (cytomegalovirus), *Toxoplasma gondii*, or human herpesviruses (HHV-6, HHV-7) can also lead to a similar syndrome.

## CLINICAL MANIFESTATIONS

IM is characterized by a combination of pharyngitis, cervical lymphadenopathy, fatigue, atypical lymphocytosis, fever, abdominal pain, and sometimes rash. There is a relatively wide range of clinically observed severity, with some patients experiencing subclinical symptomatology and others with atypical symptoms.

Pharyngitis is the most common key component of IM. Often this will be acute, with the patient reporting a moderate sore throat. On examination, tonsils are often enlarged with evidence of exudate. Exudates range in appearance, from white to gray/green/yellow in color. Palatal petechiae may also be noted. It is of course important to exclude complicating factors, such as peritonsillar abscess; however, this is relatively uncommon.

Lymphadenopathy associated with IM involves the posterior cervical chain, in contrast to predominantly anterior chain adenopathy, which is associated with streptococcal pharyngitis. The posterior cervical lymph nodes lie deep to the posterior edge of the sternocleidomastoid muscles, and require careful palpation, as they can be less obvious than enlarged anterior nodes. Lymphadenopathy with IM can, however, be diffuse, with involvement of both the anterior and cervical chains, in addition to other surrounding nodes. Lymphadenopathy is an early marker of the disease, and is often not noted until later in the clinical process, to the point that it may be resolved several weeks after symptom onset.

Rash may also be noted in the cascade of symptoms, and may present in a wide variety of ways. Often rash is diffuse, maculopapular, or petechial, and temporally associated with pharyngitis. Often, administration of beta-lactam antibiotics (most notably penicillins) can lead to a diffuse maculopapular rash in the setting of a true diagnosis of IM. This is most often seen when misdiagnosed as streptococcal pharyngitis, and can serve as a clinical indicator to consider IM.

Fatigue associated with IM can range from mild to debilitating, with many patients noting a sensation of fatigue unlike that experienced during previous respiratory illnesses. This is typically the longest-lasting symptom—in most cases fatigue lasts several weeks beyond the resolution of pharyngitis, and in some cases has been reported to last up to 6 months. It has been suggested in the literature that there is a connection between chronic fatigue syndrome (CFS) and EBV infection; however, this has not been well validated. There has been little consensus among various specialties in recent years with regard to this connection; with most agreeing that, although mononucleosis does cause acute fatigue, there have not been enough significant literature data to validate its connection to a long-term diagnosis of CFS.

The most significant finding associated with IM is the potential for hepatosplenomegaly. Although it is more common for the spleen to be involved, it is also possible that the liver may be enlarged, either on its own or simultaneously with the spleen. Some evidence has suggested that splenomegaly occurs to some degree in close to half of all cases of IM. There is much debate regarding the screening for, and management of, hepatosplenomegaly in IM, which is discussed in more detail below.

There is also the potential for associated neurologic complications, such as Guillain-Barre syndrome, or a variety of other nerve palsies. These should be carefully considered as potential complicating factors of IM.

## DIAGNOSIS

There are several methods available for the diagnosis of IM. With consideration for effective screening and economic feasibility, it is likely best to follow a stepwise approach (**Table 1**).

### Step 1

When the diagnosis of IM is suspected on the differential in an athlete based on the clinical findings discussed above, the clinician should first consider evaluating a complete blood count (CBC) with a manual differential, heterophile antibody test (Monospot); additional liver function tests may need to be considered.

In the case of IM, the CBC will often yield a lymphocytosis (absolute count >4500). The total white count is often greater than 12,000; however, this is nonspecific. Although atypical lymphocytes will often be seen on a peripheral smear, testing is not usually clinically necessary, as this finding is also not specific to IM.

There are several different heterophile antibody tests that react to different nonhuman substrates. The Monospot test is the most common, and this involves a reaction against red blood cells derived from horses. Although the Monospot remains fairly sensitive (near 85%) and specific (almost 100%), the primary issue for clinicians in the training room is the delayed time to positivity. Studies have shown that within the first week of illness there is more than a 25% false-negative rate of Monospot testing, with the rates being higher earlier in the week. In addition, heterophile antibody testing can remain positive for up to 1 year after illness.

Elevated aminotransferases are seen in most cases, and this may be of particular interest as a potential indicator of hepatic involvement when evaluating athletes.

### Step 2

Often, if the above listed testing is within the normal range, the physician can be fairly confident that IM is less likely to be the source of the athlete's symptoms. Depending on the degree of clinical suspicion, however, sometimes further testing is needed. Clinicians may simply repeat Monospot testing if clinical suspicion remains and the initial laboratory samples were drawn within the first 1 to 2 weeks. If this is negative and clinical suspicion is not extremely high, this will likely end the workup.

However, there are of course cases in which all testing is negative and clinical suspicion remains high. In these cases, it is reasonable to obtain EBV-specific antibodies

| Table 1 | | |
| --- | --- | --- |
| Suggested stepwise approach to laboratory workup for infectious mononucleosis | | |
| **Step 1 (Moderate Clinical Suspicion)** | **Step 2 (High Clinical Suspicion)** | **Further Testing Considerations** |
| • CBC with differential<br>• Heterophile antibody testing (Monospot)<br>• Liver function tests (LFTs) | • Repeat Monospot (if initial labs drawn in first 1–2 wk of illness)<br>• EBV antibodies | • Consider repeating LFTs<br>• Labs for EBV-negative IM (10% of cases): HIV antibodies, CMV antibodies, HHV-6/7, T gondii antibodies |

(**Table 2**). By obtaining the specific antibodies, the sensitivity can increase up to 97%, which is at times of vital importance in clearing an athlete.

The main antibodies tested include immunoglobulin M (IgM) and IgG antibodies against the viral capsid antigen (VCA), IgG antibody against the nuclear antigen (NA), and IgG antibody against early antigen (EA). The simplest way to understand these antibodies is to be aware that IgM and IgG antibodies against EBV-VCA are both typically present in acute IM, based on the relatively long clinical latency to illness that allows them to develop. IgM to VCA often disappears after approximately 90 days, so its presence specifically suggests acuity; whereas IgG to VCA will be present acutely, but will persist for life. On the contrary, the IgG antibody to EBV-NA does not develop until the virus establishes latency, which typically means a minimum of 6 to 12 weeks after illness. Therefore, the presence of EBV-NA essentially excludes acute illness. In addition, EBV-EA is present at the acute onset of illness in only some patients, and if present is also suggestive of acute IM. It is worth noting that the work of Pottgiesser and colleagues[1] demonstrated that EBV-EA may persist for longer than 6 months in competitive athletes, which is thought to be related to mild immunosuppression in this population, which may make this specific EBV antibody marker less helpful in athletes.

The most important factors that suggest acute illness include EBV-VCA IgM and EBV-EA, and the absence of EBV-NA. The presence of EBV-NA is critical, as its presence functionally excludes the acute diagnosis.

At this point during step 2, it is also reasonable to consider repeating liver function tests, which are abnormal in most true IM diagnoses from any origin. It can be helpful to follow downward trending values along with clinical resolution of the acute illness.

### Potential Further Testing

At this point, if concern exists for non-EBV-derived IM, further testing can be considered, because approximately 10% of IM cases are EBV negative. The alternative sources of EBV-negative IM often have additional clinical features that can help distinguish their diagnosis—which is beyond the scope of this article. Further consideration for testing includes HIV antibodies, CMV antibodies, testing for *T gondii*, and HHV-6/7.

### TREATMENT

Treating EBV-induced IM is generally supportive in nature and similar to the management of other viral syndromes. Clinicians should counsel athletes to focus on adequate rest, hydration, and nutrition. For management of pain and malaise, acetaminophen and nonsteroidal anti-inflammatory drugs are effective on an as-needed basis. Although there have been various studies, there is currently no evidence to suggest a recommendation for the use of antivirals or corticosteroids in the treatment of IM.

**Table 2**
**Summary of antibodies present in acute infectious mononucleosis compared with the antibodies that persist long term**

|  | EBV-VCA IgM | EBV-VCA IgG | EBV-NA IgG | EBV-EA IgG |
|---|---|---|---|---|
| Present in acute IM (typically) | *Yes* | Yes | *No* | Yes, sometimes |
| Present chronically with previous infection | No | Yes | Yes | No (can be present for longer periods in athletes) |

The most important factors are in italics.

## RETURN TO SPORT

The most noteworthy management topic regarding IM in athletes is the return to sport. Clinicians should follow athletes' constellation of symptoms including sore throat, fevers, and fatigue until resolution. The decision becomes more complex in the athlete who feels clinically well after a relatively short period of rest. Splenic rupture is a rare complication of IM that is at the forefront of the RTP decision, and it is of significant interest because it is potentially fatal. It is known that up to 50% of patients with the diagnosis develop hepatosplenomegaly, typically within the first 2 weeks of illness.[2] The general consensus to this point has been that most traumatic splenic ruptures tend to occur within the first 3 weeks of illness, with rare occurrences being reported all the way into the 8th week.[2-6] Based on limited case reports, most clinicians have been holding athletes back from contact sport for up to 4 to 6 weeks without any individualized screening. UpToDate recommends a minimum of 3 weeks out of sport for noncontact activity, and a minimum of 4 weeks for any contact or "strenuous" sporting activity.[7,8] Guidelines in the past have been somewhat arbitrary, without much clinical data to support the recommendations.

Some sports medicine providers have considered the possibility of using ultrasound measurement of splenomegaly specifically as a guide to individualize RTP. This is because several studies have shown a lack of reliability of physical examination (as low as 20% sensitivity) in detecting splenomegaly in this setting.[2,3,9,10] The primary problem with the use of ultrasound is the anatomic variability in the wide range of size of athletes as well as the difficulty in obtaining baseline measurements. There have been several studies attempting to outline and quantify the timing of splenomegaly in the setting of IM to guide management; however, there has been no consensus to date.

Hosey and colleagues,[3] in 2008, discussed splenomegaly as it relates to RTP for athletes, concluding that, based on 20 patients diagnosed with IM, the mean splenic length increased by 33.6%. This enlargement peaked at an average of 12.3 days from the onset of clinical symptoms, and most patients studied had resolution of splenomegaly in 4 to 6 weeks. In that study, the rate of return to normal splenic size postpeak was predictable, and they calculated it to be approximately 1% per day.

O'Connor and colleagues[11] also assessed the role of serial ultrasonography in RTP decisions. They formed a study group of 19 patients (mean age 16.7 years) diagnosed with IM. These patients were not evaluated with ultrasound at diagnosis. The investigators found that 16 out of 19 patients had normal splenic measurements on ultrasound 1 month after diagnosis, and the remaining 3 had persistent splenomegaly until the next measurement 2 months later. Their definition of normal was a spleen of 12 cm in length, 7 cm wide, and 4 cm deep—measurements based on a previous study screening 800 normal adults and finding 95% to fall in that range. If a spleen fell outside of any of those parameters, it was deemed enlarged. The obvious downside to this study was the potential for variable baseline spleen sizes confounding the results.

In an attempt to quantify this variability, a study done by Hosey and colleagues[9] in 2006 looked at splenic sizes of 631 Division 1 college athletes. Their work had several key conclusions: first, that splenic length was the most predictive measurement of volume and also the most reliable measurement between technicians; and, second, that there is likely a significant amount of variation in spleen size among individuals. Among athletes scanned, there was a range in splenic length from 5.59 to 17.06 cm observed—a discrepancy that likely should not be overlooked in reviewing the literature. This study is particularly relevant, as it specifically measured Division 1 athletes rather than adults representing much broader demographic categories.

The American Medical Society of Sports Medicine released a consensus statement in 2008 regarding IM and RTP, essentially stating that there are no evidence-based guidelines regarding the management of the condition in athletes, including RTP.[2]

To summarize, there are several factors that go into the decision to allow an athlete diagnosed with IM to RTP. Once clinical symptoms have resolved, the primary issue at hand is prevention of the potentially catastrophic outcome of splenic rupture. Based on the significant proportion of splenomegaly in IM and on the lack of case reports documenting splenic rupture in the absence of splenomegaly, it can be reasonably inferred that rupture is likely related to splenic enlargement. Based on this, clinicians may consider coordinating RTP decisions with sonographic enlargement. In our opinion, 1 possible way to guide decisions would entail obtaining a preparticipation screen of sonographic splenic measurement as a baseline. Providers may consider previous history of IM and smaller stature a way to lessen the number of athletes to screen with ultrasound. If this could be done with relative ease based on clinical resources available at the time of the preparticipation physical, it would allow for the most individualized information regarding a condition that affects up to 3% of 15- to 21-year-old athletes annually. Using this method would effectively cut out the confounding variability in splenic size between athletes. If this is not feasible in a given clinical situation, then using the gold standard baseline measurements based on the research conducted by Frank and colleagues[12,13] remains a viable approach, with splenic length being shown to have the strongest correlation with computed tomography volume assessments. If baseline splenic measurements are not obtained, several studies have demonstrated that serial ultrasounds are likely much more helpful than a single scan of an individual in determining RTP.

## REFERENCES

1. Pottgiesser T, Schumacher Y, Wolfarth B, et al. Longitudinal observation of Epstein-Barr virus antibodies in athletes during a competitive season. J Med Virol 2012;84:1415–22.
2. Putukian M, O'Connor F, Stricker P, et al. Mononucleosis and athletic participation: an evidence-based subject review. Clin J Sport Med 2008;18(4): 309–15.
3. Hosey RG, Kriss V, Uhl TL, et al. Ultrasonographic evaluation of splenic enlargement in patients with acute infectious mononucleosis. Br J Sports Med 2008;42: 974–7.
4. Bartlett A, Williams R, Hilton M. Splenic rupture in infectious mononucleosis: a systematic review of published case reports. Injury 2016;47(3):531–8.
5. Becker J, Smith JA. Return to play after infectious mononucleosis. Sports Health 2014;6(3):232–8.
6. Auwaerter PG. Infectious mononucleosis: return to play. Clin Sports Med 2004;23: 485–97.
7. Aronson M, Auwaerter P. Infectious mononucleosis. UpToDate; 2018.
8. Ebell MH. Epstein-Barr virus infectious mononucleosis. Am Fam Physician 2004; 70:1279–87.
9. Hosey RG, Mattacola CG, Kriss V, et al. Ultrasound assessment of spleen size in collegiate athletes. Br J Sports Med 2006;40:251–4.
10. Waninger KN, Harcke HT. Determination of safe return to play for athletes recovering from infectious mononucleosis: a review of the literature. Clin J Sport Med 2005;15:410–6.

11. O'Connor TE, Skinner LJ, Kiely P, et al. Return to contact sports following infectious mononucleosis: the role of serial ultrasonography. Ear Nose Throat J 2011;90(8):E21–4.
12. Frank K, Linhart P, Kortsik C, et al. Sonographic determination of spleen size: normal dimensions in adults with a healthy spleen. Ultraschall Med 1986;7(3): 134–7.
13. Spielmann AL, DeLong DM, Kliewer MA. Sonographic evaluation of spleen size in tall healthy athletes. Am J Roentgenol 2005;184:45–9.

# Common Pulmonary Conditions in Sport

Armando Gonzalez, MD*, Aaron V. Mares, MD, David R. Espinoza, MD

## KEYWORDS

- Exercise-induced bronchoconstriction (EIB) • Asthma • Respiratory infections
- Pneumothorax • Pharyngeal injury • Laryngeal injury

## KEY POINTS

- Respiratory infections present with a wide range of symptoms. Typically treated symptomatically with antitussives, expectorants, antihistamines, and nasal anti-inflammatories.
- Asthma is a chronic condition leading to airway inflammation and obstruction that is reversible with β-agonists. It can negatively affect athletes by not allowing them to compete to their full potential due to recurrence of symptoms that are exacerbated through exercise or environmental factors.
- Pneumothorax is defined as a collection of air within the pleural space between the chest wall and the lung and requires prompt recognition and treatment.
- Perforation of the pharynx or larynx can present initially with no symptoms for 24 hours to 48 hours but then develops gradually. A high index of suspicion, along with serial examinations, is required for proper diagnosis.

## RESPIRATORY INFECTIONS

Respiratory infections and their associated symptoms are common complaints among athletes and present clinically in various ways.[1–4] Typical complaints include congestion, sore throat, cough, postnasal drip, headache, fatigue, nausea, and fever. A broad differential, especially in cases of severe or nonremitting upper respiratory infection (URI) symptoms, is crucial to the recognition of potentially more serious underlying infections.

### Respiratory Infections: Work Up

Infections may be viral or bacterial in etiology, with a majority of cases being viral. Various etiologies for a URI include sinusitis, pharyngitis, peritonsillar abscess, lower respiratory infection, bronchitis, and pneumonia. A diagnosis is made primarily

---

Disclosure: We as authors of this article have no commercial or financial conflicts of interest or any funding sources that may conflict with the writing of this article.
Department of Orthopaedics, The University of Pittsburgh, 3200 South Water Street, Pittsburgh, PA 15203, USA
* Corresponding author.
E-mail address: mandogonzalezmd@gmail.com

Clin Sports Med 38 (2019) 563–575
https://doi.org/10.1016/j.csm.2019.06.005
0278-5919/19/© 2019 Elsevier Inc. All rights reserved.

through history and physical examination, and most of these illnesses do not require extensive work-up. In the presence of systemic symptoms or red flag symptoms, however, such as lethargy, confusion, or worsening quality of symptoms, it may be necessary to rule out other potential causes. Laboratory work-up may include a complete blood cell count, blood chemistries, viral screening, Epstein-Barr virus titers, throat culture, and, for the presence of lower respiratory symptoms and examination findings, a chest radiograph.

### Respiratory Infections: Treatment

Viral URIs can be treated symptomatically with over-the-counter medications, such as antihistamines, decongestants, and vitamin supplementation, such as vitamin C and zinc. Most viral-induced URIs typically resolve within 1 week but can last for up to 10 days to 14 days with continued cough. If an athlete presents with systemic symptoms, such as fever, tachycardia, hypoxia, or respiratory distress, the etiology may be bacterial. Athletes who have positive sputum and blood cultures or have a chest radiograph showing a pulmonary infiltrate in the presence of systemic symptoms have a higher likelihood of having a bacterial etiology. Initiation of proper antibiotic is necessary and should be chosen based on the likely pathogen. Dehydration is a common sequela of such significant respiratory infections due to increased insensible water loss; athletes should be counseled on maintaining adequate hydration and caloric intake as a critical part of their recuperation. Aggressive supportive measures may need to be implemented depending on illness severity.

### Respiratory Infections: Return to Play

Return-to-sport decisions should be made on an individual basis, with close follow-up and monitoring. If an athlete engages in sport with a fever greater than 101°F, there is an increased risk of developing myocarditis. The athlete should be held from participation until the fever resolves, without the use of any antipyretic, for a period of 24 hours. It also is important to rule out infectious mononucleosis with its risk for splenic enlargement and possible splenic rupture. Athletes diagnosed with mononucleosis, confirmed with Epstein-Barr virus titers for an acute infection, should be held out from play in contact sport for at least 3 weeks from the onset of symptoms (see dedicated Anthony S. Ceraulo and Jeffrey R. Bytomski's article, "Infectious Mononucleosis in the Training Room," in this issue to infectious mononucleosis in this edition).

There are no clear return-to-play guidelines when it comes to a URI. For symptoms that are upper respiratory in nature (neck up), such as sore throat, nasal congestion, or sinusitis, without other systemic involvement, an athlete may be cleared to participate. If there are lower respiratory tract symptoms along with systemic symptoms (neck down), such as fever or myalgia, then it is prudent for the athlete to be held from participation until symptoms resolve due to risk of myocarditis and other fatigue-induced injury.

## ASTHMA

Asthma is a chronic pulmonary condition characterized by airway inflammation, hyper-responsiveness, and reversible airway obstruction that can negatively affect athletes to varying degrees. The prevalence of respiratory symptoms and disease tends to be higher in athletes compared with the general population. The prevalence of asthma varies with respect to training environment and may involve up to 50% of athletes, depending on the sport environment. The prevalence of exercise-induced bronchoconstriction (EIB) is even higher, with a range of 30% to 70% among athletes.[5]

## Asthma: Pathophysiology

In asthmatics, a chronic inflammatory state of the lungs leads to increased levels of cytokines and inflammatory molecules within the bronchial tree, resulting in airway narrowing and obstruction. When exposed to certain triggers, an inflammatory cascade produces increased mucus that leads to edema of the bronchial epithelium and bronchial muscle constriction. Triggers and antigens include pollen, mold, allergens, cold air, and even exercise itself.

## Asthma: Symptoms and Presentation

Athletes may present with symptoms of cough, wheezing, dyspnea, phlegm production, or chest tightness. Symptoms can progress to life-threatening hypoxia due to lower airway obstruction. A diagnosis of asthma typically is made by history and physical examination, with episodes of dyspnea associated with certain triggers—at times a patient diary may be of benefit to pinpoint these triggers because it is important to identify them for best long-term control of asthma.

## Asthma: Diagnosis

Empiric treatment with a short-acting $\beta$-agonist (SABA) inhaler (albuterol or equivalent) that resolves symptoms is a common way to make a diagnosis of asthma. Pulmonary function testing with spirometry can be used to diagnose this condition objectively. Spirometry is a functional test used to objectively diagnose asthma and measures the following variables: forced expiratory volume in 1 second ($FEV_1$), as the athlete forcibly exhales with the volume of air measured over 1 second, and forced vital capacity (FVC), where the volume of air is measured on full exhalation after taking a full inhalation. If the ratio of $FEV_1$/FVC is less than 70%, along with $FEV_1$ being less than 80% predicted, then asthma may be the diagnosis. The diagnosis is confirmed via reversibility of $FEV_1$ with an increase of greater than 12% from baseline or greater than or equal to 10% of the predicted $FEV_1$ after use of a SABA inhaler. Based on history and spirometry results, the diagnosis of asthma can be classified into categories dependent on the severity of disease (**Table 1**).

**Table 1**
**Diagnosis criterion for levels of asthma severity**

| | Impairment | | | Risk | |
|---|---|---|---|---|---|
| Severity Category | Days and Nights with Symptoms | Interference with Normal Activity | Pulmonary Function | Exacerbations | Preferred Treatment |
| Severe Persistent | Throughout (d) Often, 7×/wk (nights) | Extremely limited | $FEV_1$: <60% $FEV_1$/FVC: reduced >5% | 2 or more/y | Step 5: high-dose ICS + LABA and consider short-course OCS Step 4: medium-dose ICS + LABA and consider short-course OCS |

(continued on next page)

**Table 1**
*(continued)*

| Severity Category | Days and Nights with Symptoms | Interference with Normal Activity | Pulmonary Function | Exacerbations | Preferred Treatment |
|---|---|---|---|---|---|
| | | **Impairment** | | **Risk** | |
| Moderate Persistent | Daily (d) 2–6 nights/wk (nights) | Some limitation | $FEV_1$: 60% to 80% $FEV_1$/FVC: reduced 5% | 2 or more/y | Step 3: low-dose ICS + LABA OR Medium-dose ICS and consider short-course OCS |
| Mild Persistent | 3–6 d/wk (d) 3–4 nights/mo (nights) | Minor limitation | $FEV_1$: >80% $FEV_1$/FVC: normal | 2 or more/y | Step 2: low-dose ICS |
| Interminent | ≤2 d/wk (d) ≤2 nights/mo (nights) | None | $FEV_1$: >80% $FEV_1$/FVC: normal | 0–1/y | Step 1: SABA prn |

*Abbreviations:* ICS, inhaled corticosteroids; OCS, oral corticosteroids.
*Adapted from* the National Asthma Education and Prevention Program. *Expert Panel Report 3: Guidelines for the Diagnosis and management of Asthma, 2007.* NIH Publication No. 07-4051. Bethesda, Md: National Heart, Lung, and Blood Institute; 2007.

## Asthma: Treatment

Treating asthma relies on 3 key components: medication management focused on prevention of symptoms, education and knowledge of triggers and medication compliance, and creating an action plan in case of an acute asthma exacerbation. Athletes must be knowledgeable of the proper indications for and usage of their SABA, along with compliance of their preventative medications. Identification of triggers for symptoms is a key component of treatment; these may include seasonal allergies, environmental antigens, weather changes, or even URIs. An individual must demonstrate vigilance to keep symptoms under control by altering environmental exposures and maintaining structured, regular use of medications. These environmental changes may include changing practice locations based on the weather, using a humidifier or antiallergen air filters at home, or even avoiding the use of nonsteroidal anti-inflammatory drugs, because they may predispose athletes to asthma flares.[6,7] Athletes and athletic trainers should be aware and be reminded to rely on their asthma action plan provided by their primary care physician that demonstrates a step-by-step process of what to do when their symptoms begin to become uncontrolled (**Figs. 1** and **2**).

The athlete, physician, and athletic trainer should be aware of symptom presentation variability and be alert for symptoms suggesting a frank exacerbation. Important and relevant past medical history include date of last exacerbation, date of last hospitalization, if the athlete has ever needed to be transferred to a facility for a higher level of care, and if the patient has ever been intubated and mechanically ventilated. Peak flows also may be utilized to monitor severity of asthma symptoms; however, compliance among the athletic population may be problematic.

When it comes to treatment of asthma in elite athletes who* are subjected to banned substance testing, it is vital that athletes and medical staff are aware of governing body guidelines. For example, the World Anti-Doping Agency guidelines prohibit the use of all inhaled β-agonists, except salmeterol, salbutamol (1600 µg maximum over 24 hours), and formoterol (54 µg maximum over 24 hours).[8] Medical personnel must be aware of the list of banned substances when it comes to caring for elite athletes participating in Olympic or professional-level events.

---

## Asthma Action Plan

**AMERICAN LUNG ASSOCIATION.**

Name _____ DOB ___/___/___

**Severity Classification** ☐ Intermittent ☐ Mild Persistent ☐ Moderate Persistent ☐ Severe Persistent

**Asthma Triggers** (list) _____

**Peak Flow Meter Personal Best** _____

### Green Zone: Doing Well

**Symptoms:** Breathing is good – No cough or wheeze – Can work and play – Sleeps well at night

**Peak Flow Meter** _____ (more than 80% of personal best)

| Control Medicine(s) | Medicine | How much to take | When and how often to take it |
|---|---|---|---|
| | _____ | _____ | _____ |
| | _____ | _____ | _____ |

**Physical Activity** ☐ Use albuterol/levalbuterol _____ puffs, 15 min before activity
☐ with all activity ☐ when you feel you need it

### Yellow Zone: Caution

**Symptoms:** Some problems breathing – Cough, wheeze, or chest tight – Problems working or playing – Wake at night

**Peak Flow Meter** _____ to _____ (between 50% and 79% of personal best)

**Quick-relief** Medicine(s) ☐ Albuterol/levalbuterol _____ puffs, every 4 h as needed

**Control Medicine(s)** ☐ Continue Green Zone medicines
☐ Add _____ ☐ Change to _____

You should feel better within 20–60 min of the quick-relief treatment. If you are getting worse or are in the Yellow Zone for more than 24 h, THEN follow the instructions in the RED ZONE and call the doctor right away!

### Red Zone: Get Help Now!

**Symptoms:** Lots of problems breathing – Cannot work or play – Getting worse instead of better – Medicine is not helping

**Peak Flow Meter** _____ (less than 50% of personal best)

**Take Quick-relief Medicine NOW!** ☐ Albuterol/levalbuterol _____ puffs, _____ (how frequently)

**Call 911 immediately if the following danger signs are present** • Trouble walking/talking due to shortness of breath
• Lips or fingernails are blue
• Still in the red zone after 15 min

**Emergency Contact** Name _____ Phone (_____) _____-_____
**Healthcare Provider** Name _____ Phone (_____) _____-_____

1-800-LUNGUSA | LUNG.org

Date ___/___/___

**Fig. 1.** Asthma action plan from American Lung Association. (*Courtesy of* American Lung Association. Learn more at Lung.org/asthma.)

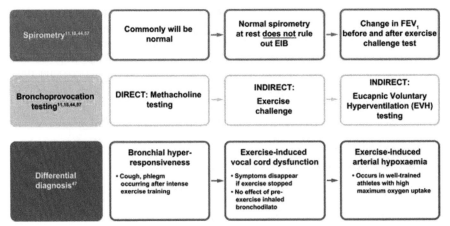

**Fig. 2.** Algorithm for diagnosis of asthma. (*From* Arrarwal, Mulgirigama, Berend, N (2018) Exercise-induced bronchoconstriction: prevalence, pathophysiology, patient impact, diagnosis, and management. NPJ Primary Care Respiratory Medicine 28.31; with permission.)

## Asthma: Return to Play

It is acceptable to allow an athlete to return to sport once symptoms abate and pulmonary function tests return to baseline. With appropriate treatment, medications generally result in more rapid improvement of symptoms and allow the athlete to return to sport more quickly.

## EXERCISE-INDUCED BRONCHOCONSTRICTION

EIB is a pulmonary condition characterized by transient reversible airway narrowing that increases respiratory resistance resulting in coughing, shortness of breath, wheezing, or chest tightness shortly after vigorous exercise. EIB can occur in athletes with and without asthma. The symptoms of EIB can significantly increase performance anxiety due to increased fearfulness, frustration, and embarrassment compared with those without symptoms.[9]

### Exercise-induced Bronchoconstriction: Symptoms and Presentation

EIB is a condition distinct from asthma that typically presents after 5 minutes to 10 minutes of vigorous exercise and can last up to 20 minutes to 30 minutes after exercise has concluded.[6] Symptoms that are reversible and do not occur at rest are pathognomonic for EIB. An athlete can present with a variety of symptoms, such as breathlessness, chest congestion, tightness, postexercise cough, fatigue, or wheezing.[10-12] Atypical symptoms include stomach cramps, chest pain, headache, recurrent cough, and phlegm production.[10] Symptoms also may be influenced by other factors, including weather, allergens, and intermittent bursts of exercise intensity during match play.[13]

### Exercise-induced Bronchoconstriction: Pathophysiology

There are 2 main theories as to the pathophysiology of EIB: thermal expenditure and osmotic. The thermal expenditure theory states that airway cooling during the increased respiratory rate of sport activity causes vasoconstriction of the lower airway bronchial tree. Subsequently, the rewarming of the airway leads to dilation of the vasculature leading to vascular leakage and edema.[14] The increase in ventilation, in particular in cold weather environments, can further lead to dehydration of the airway surfaces, causing changes in bronchial blood flow. Cold weather events, such as skiing and ice hockey, demonstrate the highest rates of EIB.[9]

Hyperventilation during exercise leads to transient osmotic changes at the airway surface, which triggers mast cell degranulation. When there is a mast cell–mediated release, there is a release of signaling molecules (prostaglandins, leukotrienes, histamine, and tryptase) known to mediate airway smooth muscle contraction, increase mucus production, increase microvascular permeability, and increase sensory nerve activation, which is thought to be the main stimulus for bronchoconstriction and airway edema.[9]

With normal function, the bronchial system warms air prior to it reaching the lower airway; however, in EIB there is inadequate temperature regulation of the air by the upper airway system before that air reaches the lower airway and bronchial tree. While at rest, the upper airway's ability to warm the air is permissible due to a slower respiratory rate. During exertion, the respiratory rate increases, allowing less time for the cool environmental air to be warmed prior to reaching the lower airways. The distal bronchial tree then comes in contact with colder air than usual, which results in an athlete's symptoms of EIB due to the mechanisms, described previously.

## Exercise-induced Bronchoconstriction: Diagnosis

Diagnosis of EIB typically is made through history and physical examination. The difficulty with objectively diagnosing EIB, however, is due to the spectrum of symptom severity and presentation. EIB should be considered when patients report symptoms that are induced by exercise.[9] To properly diagnose this condition, pulmonary function tests should be conducted while at rest to evaluate for any underlying chronic asthma. Then, ideally, pulmonary function tests would be obtained after exercise(s) that provoke symptoms.[9] Evidence of an exercise-induced decrease in expiratory volume establishes the diagnosis, as discussed later. In some circumstances, an empiric trial of a SABA may be used; if symptoms resolve with use, then this could be diagnostic of EIB in the proper setting. Should a diagnosis not make itself evident, other pathologies should be ruled out, including vocal cord dysfunction, gastroesophageal reflux, and cardiac abnormalities. Some individuals may present with a refractory period, where in the time after the resolution of symptoms the athletes do not experience any further exacerbations for the next 1 hour to 2 hours; however, they may have return of symptoms after this time period.[6]

A diagnosis of EIB can be made with the following: an exercise challenge test, eucapnic voluntary hyperventilation (EVH) test, hyperosmolar saline challenge test, mannitol challenge test, or direct challenge test with the use of methacholine to induce bronchoconstriction. The most commonly used tests are the exercise challenge test and the EVH test. These tests focus on the $FEV_1$ and its decline from baseline after provocation. A decline in $FEV_1$ great than 10% in EVH test or peak expiratory flow rate of 15% or greater indicate positive results with these tests.[6,13]

## Exercise-induced Bronchoconstriction: Treatment

The treatment of EIB is different with a patient who has a known history of asthma as opposed to an individual who does not have asthma. In athletes without asthma, management of EIB should focus on relief of bronchoconstriction and modification of risk factors. The goal is to allow the patient to continue to engage in activity with minimal respiratory symptoms.[9] Nonpharmacologic approaches are first-line treatment of EIB and include prewarmed, humidified inhaled air during exercise (ie, breathing through a face mask) and avoiding exposure to allergens.[9] Pharmacologic treatment of these athletes is similar to the acute treatment of an athlete with asthma and is discussed in the next few sections. In athletes who present with EIB superimposed on a history of baseline asthma, the primary goal of management is to ensure that the underlying asthma is well controlled.

Many of the same medications used to treat chronic asthma can be utilized for EIB as well; 2 puffs to 4 puffs of a SABA inhaler, such as albuterol 20 minutes prior to exercise, often controls or prevents the onset of symptoms. Although the use of a SABA prior to activity is strongly recommended, the daily use of SABA has shown to lead to tolerance and therefore ideally should be used to prevent EIB on an intermittent basis only.[15] Inhaled corticosteroids do not play a role in the management and treatment of EIB, but they do need to be used in the management of the athlete who presents with EIB symptoms superimposed on a history of asthma.

In patients with EIB and asthma, the American Thoracic Society recommends the use of inhaled corticosteroids, even though their onset of maximal improvement typically lasts 2 weeks to 4 weeks.[9] The main issue to address is improvement of suboptimally controlled asthma. For patients who continue to have symptoms, despite the use of inhaled SABA before exercise or require more frequent use, the daily use of a of long-acting $\beta_2$-agonist (LABA) should only be considered in conjunction with inhaled corticosteroid use. LABA as a single therapy is not recommended due to known associations with acute exacerbations. If EIB does not respond to SABA therapy, mast cell stabilizers also may be recommended.[9]

With regard to treatment of EIB, it is important to look at all modifiable factors as well as pharmacologic options. The use of scarves or masks can limit the amount of cool air that reaches the lower respiratory tract, theoretically decreasing the trigger for bronchoconstriction. A short warm-up period 15 minutes to 20 minutes prior to activity at 80% to 90% of maximum exertion and proper cool-downs postexertion have been shown to limit the EIB response in athletes.[16]

### Exercise-induced Bronchoconstriction: Return to Play

An athlete experiencing dyspneic symptoms should be removed from play and evaluated properly on the sideline. If a baseline spirometry is known, repeat testing at the time of symptom onset should be conducted to assist in the evaluation of symptom severity.[16] If the spirometry is below 15% from baseline, then 2 puffs of a SABA may be given with another 2 puffs if symptoms are still present after 5 minutes.[16] Serial spirometry readings can be conducted until the value returns to normal limits or back to baseline. If values do not return to normal or baseline, then the athlete should be evaluated for other potential causes and treatments, including emergency options as the condition could progress to a life-threatening state, such as status asthmaticus.[16] Once athletes' respiratory function has improved and they are no longer symptomatic, they may return to the playing field.

## VOCAL CORD DYSFUNCTION AND EXERCISE-INDUCED LARYNGEAL OBSTRUCTION

In the presentation of asthma and EIB-like symptoms that do not respond to management as expected, a differential diagnosis of exercise-induced laryngeal obstruction (EILO) should be considered. EILO encompasses a variety of disorders that lead to abnormal function of the vocal cords within the larynx during exercise. This complex network of muscle and cartilaginous structures with unique neurologic input functions to prevent aspiration of food during swallowing, prevent inhalation of noxious substances during respiration, and produce voice and sound with respiration.[17] The mucosal lining of the larynx contains multiple receptors that are affected by various factors, including temperature, pressure, tracheal movement, and environmental irritants, and, when this delicate homeostasis is disrupted by any one of these factors, it can lead to dysfunction of the vocal cords and laryngeal obstruction with exercise. EILO can manifest as a result of laryngeal hyperresponsiveness and psychogenic and neurogenic disorders as well as laryngeal irritation from viral respiratory illness, gastroesophageal reflux, cold temperatures, postnasal drip with allergies, and even exposure to sudden strong odors.[17]

The prevalence of EILO is difficult to discern due to its high concomitance with EIB (>50%) and asthma (56%), but some studies report that it affects up to 5% to 7% of the adolescent population, with a higher incidence among women and the athletic population, in particular those participating in outdoor sports.[17,18] Presentation of EILO can be similar to that of EIB, with the main symptom of shortness of breath and dyspnea at the close of exercise and up to 2 minutes to 3 minutes after exercise. EILO can be differentiated from EIB and asthma by the presence of harsh inspiratory stridor with auscultation and a prolonged inspiratory phase as opposed to EIB and asthma that demonstrate expiratory wheezing with a prolonged expiratory phase.[18] Due to symptom similarity, acute episodes often are treated with inhaled bronchodilators that may help with the concomitant bronchospasm but do little to help with the vocal cord dysfunction.[17]

The gold-standard diagnostic test for EILO is a continuous laryngoscopy exercise test because it allows for direct feedback and visualization of the vocal cords during an acute event with provocation of symptoms.[18] Pulmonary function tests and even trial treatments with EIB and asthma medications, however, can help lead to the diagnosis of EILO. Treatment and management also tends to be complex due to the multitude of factors that affect the larynx; therefore, a multidisciplinary approach is needed for proper identification and management, as demonstrated in **Table 2**.

**Table 2**
**Management of vocal cord dysfunction based on etiology**

| Referral | Work-up | Diagnosis | Comment |
|---|---|---|---|
| Pulmonology | Pulmonary function tests ± exercise challenged | Identify comorbid EIB or other pulmonary disease | Shortened inspiratory flow-volume loop |
| Otolaryngology | Laryngoscopy ± exercise challenge to assess structure and function for possible sources of compression/ obstruction | Anatomic stenosis vs extrinsic compression Rule out airway obstruction Inflammatory causes of compression Vocal cord dysfunction | Coexisting GERD may contribute to symptoms Differential diagnosis of GERD vs allergic rhinitis, with appropriate treatment |
| Speech- language pathology | VCD management and training | Via laryngoscopy | Techniques to tighten/ relax, diaphragmatic breathing, breathing recover |
| Psychiatry/ behavioral health | Identify coexisting depression, anxiety, OCD | Identification of psychological stressors contributing to VCD | Pharmacotherapy Behavioral management |
| Allergy and immunology | Allergy testing | Identify specific environmental allergens | Pharmacotherapy Exposure avoidance |

*Abbreviations:* GERD, gastroesophageal reflux disease; OCD obsessive compulsive disorder; VCD, vocal cord dysfunction.

## PNEUMOTHORAX

A pneumothorax (PTX) is defined as a collection of air within the pleural space between the chest wall and the lung. This is a potentially life-threatening condition that requires prompt recognition and treatment. Due to the negative intrathoracic pressure created by inspiration, the accumulation of this air can eventually reach high enough pressures to collapse the lung, leading to cardiopulmonary compromise. Pneumothoraces can be spontaneous or tension related, and only 2% of all adult pneumothoraces are associated with sports.[19,20]

Spontaneous PTX is often found in young, tall, thin individuals. Primary spontaneous PTX typically happens suddenly and without insult, whereas secondary PTX typically occurs in the setting of underlying pulmonary disease, such as pneumonia, asthma, cystic fibrosis, or interstitial lung disease. Tension PTX is much less common and typically occurs due to disruption of the lung pleura secondary to blunt or penetrating trauma from a fractured rib that disrupts the pleura.

### Pneumothorax: Symptoms and Presentation

Signs and symptoms include difficulty breathing, pleuritic pain on inspiration, increased respiratory rates, and tachycardia. These symptoms often are progressive; performing serial physical examinations and vital sign checks is crucial to early recognition and diagnosis of this pathology. After blunt trauma; associated conditions, such as pulmonary contusion, hemothorax, pneumo-mediastinum, splenic rupture, kidney laceration, rib fracture, or other internal derangement, must be recognized and excluded.

### Pneumothorax: Diagnosis

Serial examinations are essential in monitoring the evolution of a PTX. Onset can be gradual or acute with potential cardiopulmonary compromise. The pulmonary examination may include diminished breath sounds, rales, hyperresonance on percussion, tachycardia, hypoxia, hypotension. Tension PTX may result in tracheal deviation away from the affected side. Thoracic wall injury, including rib fractures and cardiac involvement, must be excluded as concurrent diagnoses.

Imaging should include a chest radiograph as the first-line modality of choice. Ultrasound can also be useful as well but may be limited by user experience and technique. CT imaging can be utilized once a patient is stabilized to assess for any associated pathology, such as pulmonary contusion, organ laceration, or rib fractures. Once a diagnosis is even suspected, the transport of the athlete to a nearby emergency department for higher-level care, evaluation, and treatment is necessary due to risk of respiratory compromise and overall decompensation. A high index of suspicion for PTX is required after blunt trauma that leads to the development of respiratory symptoms or limited physical exertion.

### Pneumothorax: Treatment

Depending on PTX size, treatment of an uncomplicated PT may be observational with serial chest radiographs until resolution. An example of this is a no-tension PTX less than 10%. The American College of Chest Physicians recommends that a small PTX (<3 cm apex-to-cupola distance) in a hemodynamically stable patient, without significant symptoms, may be managed by observation alone with close follow-up after the exclusion of progression. They are typically observed for 3 hours to 6 hours with a repeat chest radiograph in an emergency setting. Larger pneumothoraces (>3 cm) should be re-expanded with chest tube decompression.[21]

Should a tension PTX be suspected, the athlete is to be given supplemental oxygen for respiratory support, and needle decompression with either a 14-gauge or larger needle can be performed. The needle is inserted along the midclavicular line into the second intercostal space to relieve the pressure, which may or may not be followed by a rush of air.[21] This is subsequently followed by placement of a chest tube to allow for lung re-expansion. Repeat chest radiograph to visualize re-expansion of the lung and ensure proper chest tube placement is recommended, then followed by serial chest radiographs, a minimum of 2 days later, to ensure stability. If the PTX remains resolved, the chest tube can be removed after 2 days to 3 days of monitoring in an acute care setting.

### Pneumothorax: Return to Play

There is no set of universal consensus guidelines when it comes to return to play after a PTX. Air travel should be avoided in the first 1 week to 3 weeks after a PTX as the change in air pressure may result in gas expansion in a closed parenchymal space leading to hypoxemia. There are no consensus data, however, to suggest an optimal time to fly after a PTX. During this time, repeat chest radiograph should be obtained to ensure continued resolution of the PTX, along with symptomatic treatment that may include beta-agonists, mucolytics, and cough suppressants for patient comfort. A chest wall protector may also be implemented for extra protection depending on the sport.

Close follow-up should also be implemented to ensure that the development of acute respiratory distress syndrome does not occur.

## PHARYNGEAL AND LARYNGEAL TRAUMA

Perforation of the pharynx or larynx is fortunately rather rare in sport. Clinically there may be no symptoms for 24 hours to 48 hours followed then by insidious onset of sore throat, neck pain, dysphagia, or excessive expectoration of saliva, which may progress to feelings of pressure in the throat and discernible swelling on examination. Serial examiantions and close monitoring along with a high index of suspicion typically are required for proper diagnosis. Initial testing typically begins with cervical radiogrpahs that are followed by CT with intravenous contrast, barium

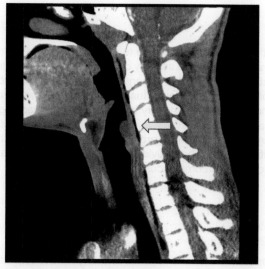

**Fig. 3.** Sagittal CT with retropharyngeal emphysema, as demonstrated by the yellow arrow.

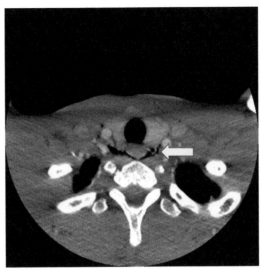

**Fig. 4.** Axial CT with retropharyngeal emphysema, as demonstrated by yellow arrow.

swallow, and laryngoscopy in order to confirm the diagnosis, as shown in **Figs. 3 and 4.**

Once a diagnosis is made, treatment is based on the size and location of perforation. In general, perforations less than 2 cm can be treated nonoperatively; however, if the perforation extends into the esophagus or is larger than 2 cm, surgical intervention is often required. Nonoperative treatment is centered around empiric treatment with antibiotics, avoidance of coughing, sneezing, or vomiting, and gradual progression with oral tolerance of liquids, soft foods, and then regular foods. Follow-up advanced imaging also is required to ensure resolution of pathology. Return-to-play criteria are not clear-cut. Resolution of pathology by imaging and symptoms typically is used as a guide to determining safety to return to activity.

## SUMMARY

Pulmonary conditions present a challenge to a sports medicine team given the spectrum of disorders and the potential severity of their associated symptoms. History and physical examination help establish a diagnosis as well as help recognize potential emergent situations. In nonemergent situations, peak flow measurements, environment exposure management, pulmonary conditioning, pharmacologic management, and action plans are useful modalities. In emergent situations, assessment of airway, breathing, and circulation as well as prompt diagnosis is critical. It is stressed that return-to-play criteria should be individualized, with recommendations depending on an athlete's individual circumstances.

## REFERENCES

1. Allen TW. Return to play following exercise-induced bronchoconstriction. Clin J Sports Med 2005;15(6):421–5.

2. Ansley L, Kippelen P, Dickinson J, et al. Misdiagnosis of exercise-induced bronchoconstriction in professional soccer players. Allergy 2011;67:390–5.

3. Boulet LP, Turmel J, Cote A. Asthma and exercise-induced respiratory symptoms in the athlete: New insights. Curr Opin Pulm Med 2017;23(1):71–7.
4. Feden JP. Closed lung trauma. Clin Sports Med 2013;32:255–65.
5. Boulet L-P, Turmel J, Côté A, et al. Asthma and exercise-induced respiratory symptoms in the athlete: new insights. Curr Opin Pulm Med 2017;23(1):71–7.
6. Lazovic B, Mazic S, Suzic-Lazic J, et al. Respiratory adaptations in different types of sport. Eur Rev Med Pharmacol Sci 2015;19:2269–74.
7. Mead WF, Harwig R. Fitness evaluation and exercise prescription. J Fam Pract 1981;13(7):1039–50.
8. Hull JH, Ansley L, Robson-Ansley P, et al. Managing respiratory problems in athletes. Clin Med 2012;12(4):351–6.
9. Arrarwal M, Berend N. Exercise-induced bronchoconstriction: prevalence, pathophysiology, patient impact, diagnosis, and management. NPJ Prim Care Respir Med 2018;28:31.
10. Brennan FH Jr, Alent J, Ross MJ, et al. Evaluated the athlete with suspected exercise-induced asthma or bronchospasm. Curr Sports Med Rep 2018;17(3):85–9.
11. Wood P, Hill V. Practical management of asthma. Pediatr Rev 2009;30:10.
12. American Lung Association. Create an asthma action plan. Available at: https://www.lung.org/lung-health-and-diseases/lung-disease-lookup/asthma/living-with-asthma/managing-asthma/create-an-asthma-action-plan.html. Accessed October 17, 2018.
13. Jaworski CA. Pulmonary. In: O'Connor FG, Casa DJ, Davis BA, et al, editors. ACSM's sports medicine: a comprehensive review, vol. 38. 1st edition. New York: Wolters-Kluwer LIppincott Williams & Wilkins; 2013. p. 248–55.
14. Partridge R, Coley A, Bowie R, et al. Sports-related pneumothorax. Ann Emerg Med 1997;30(4):539–41.
15. Parsons JP, Hallstrand TS, Mastronarde JG, et al. An official American Thoracic Society Clinical practice guideline: exercise-induced bronchoconstriction. Am J Respir Crit Care Med 2013;187:1016–27.
16. Pongdee T, James TL. Exercise-induced bronchoconstriction. Ann Allergy Asthma Immunol 2013;110:311–5.
17. Wilson JJ, Theis SM, Wilson EM. Evaluation and management of vocal cord dysfunction in the athlete. Curr Sports Med Rep 2009;8(2):65–70.
18. Liyanagedara S, McLeod R, Elhassan H. exercise induced laryngeal obstruction: a review of diagnosis and management. Eur Arch Otorhinolaryngol 2017;274:1781–9.
19. Weiler JM, Bonini S, Coifman R, et al, Ad Hoc Committee of Sports Medicine Committee of American Academy of Allergy, Asthma & Immunology. American academy of allergy, asthma and immunology work group report: exercise-induced asthma. J Allergy Clin Immunol 2007;119(6):1349–58.
20. What is asthma? National heart lung and blood institute NIH. 2014. Available at: https://www.nhlbi.nih.gov. Accessed October 17, 2018.
21. What is prohibited. World Anti-Doping Agency. 2016. Available at: https://www.wada-ama.org/en/prohibited-list. Accessed October 17, 2018.

# Acute Illness in the Athlete

Carrie A. Jaworski, MD[a,b],*, Valerie Rygiel, DO[c]

## KEYWORDS

- Acute illness • Infectious disease • Pertussis • Influenza • Travelers diarrhea
- Urinary tract infection • Sexually transmitted disease

## KEY POINTS

- Athletes are susceptible to many acute illnesses that can interfere with their ability to train and compete as well as potentially affecting teammates and coaching staff.
- A solid understanding of the preventive measures, diagnosis, and management of such diseases is paramount in the care of an athletic population.

Acute illnesses contracted by athletes typically mirror the type and timing of those seen in the general population; however, in athletes they can present as a significant health burden. When caring for acutely ill athletes, sports medicine providers need to consider how the illness can affect the athlete's training, performance, and competition schedule; the risk of transmission of the illness to other team members; and the necessary precautions and contraindications related to treatment of the athletes and their return to participation. In addition, it is necessary to recognize that athletes training at an elite level, or for more prolonged periods of time, may be more susceptible to illness as a facet of an overtraining syndrome. This article focuses on the impact of acute illness on athletes as well as highlighting special considerations of specific acute illnesses as they relate to athletes.

## THE RELATIONSHIP BETWEEN EXERCISE AND IMMUNE FUNCTION

The proposed effects of exercise on immune function have typically been poorly understood. The literature supports both the positive and negative effects that exercise can have on immune function and risk of illness.[1–3] The risk of illness has been found to increase in situations of prolonged and/or intense training, especially in athletes who are already immunocompromised, have high levels of intrinsic or extrinsic stressors, or have had a recent infection.[4] However, most athletes training at a moderate level

[a] Division of Primary Care Sports Medicine, NorthShore University HealthSystem, Glenview, IL, USA; [b] Department of Family Medicine, University of Chicago, Pritzker School of Medicine, Chicago, IL, USA; [c] Primary Care Sports Medicine Fellowship, University of Chicago/NorthShore University HealthSystem, 2180 Pfingsten Road, Suite 3100, Glenview, IL 60026, USA
* Corresponding author. University of Chicago/NorthShore University HealthSystem Primary Care Sports Medicine Fellowship, 2180 Pfingsten Road, Suite 3100, Glenview, IL 60026.
E-mail address: CJaworski@NorthShore.org

Clin Sports Med 38 (2019) 577–595
https://doi.org/10.1016/j.csm.2019.05.001
0278-5919/19/© 2019 Elsevier Inc. All rights reserved.

benefit from improved immune function and lower infection rates compared with people who do not exercise.

Several theories have been proposed in the literature with regard to exercise and immune function, with the 2 most widely accepted being the J-curve model and the open-window theory. The J-curve model is based on evidence that moderate exercise enhances immune function compared with that of sedentary individuals, whereas excessive, intense exercise may paradoxically impair immune function.[2] This theory is generally accepted as true except in the case of elite, international-level, and medal-winning athletes, in whom high training levels do not impart a negative effect on performance.[5–7] The reasons for this are unclear, but are thought to be related to self-selection, whereby this group of athletes possess immune systems able to withstand the highest levels of physiologic and psychological stressors, which results in what is referred to as an S-curve phenomenon[8] (**Fig. 1**).

The open-window theory proposes that the immune system is temporarily downregulated for a period of time after strenuous exercise, leading to a window in which the risk of infection increases. The depressive effect on immune function can last between 3 and 24 hours after exercise, depending on intensity and duration of the exercise, with greater suppression seen with more intense and prolonged bouts of exercise[9] (**Fig. 2**).

Despite these theories, there is limited evidence that showing a direct correlation between exercise-induced impaired immune function and an increased incidence of clinically confirmed infection.[1]

## ILLNESS AND PERFORMANCE

Acute illnesses in athletes stand to affect performance through a variety of mechanisms. Infections occurring during the peak of an athlete's season can impair the athlete's competitive performance because of being limited by symptoms, such as with a persistent cough, as well as via deconditioning from lost training time. In contrast, an infection early in the season is less likely to impart significant consequences because any decline in performance can typically be regained quickly once the illness resolves. Respiratory symptoms such as cough and bronchospasm can directly affect ventilation and aerobic capacity as well as incite anxiety in the athlete because of either a real

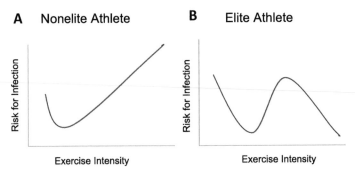

## The J and S Hypothesis

**A**  Nonelite Athlete      **B**  Elite Athlete

**Fig. 1.** (*A*) In nonelite athletes, moderate amounts of exercise decrease the risk for infections, whereas excessive intense exercise increases the risk. (*B*) Elite athletes are not susceptible to the same negative effect.

# The Open-window Hypothesis

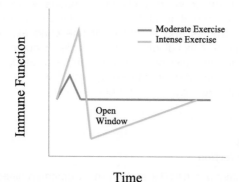

**Fig. 2.** The immune system is temporarily downregulated after exercise, leading to a window where in which risk of infection increases.

or perceived inability to oxygenate properly. Fever impairs the ability to regulate body temperature, which increases fluid losses and can affect both stroke volume and cardiac output, affecting maximal oxygen uptake ($Vo_{2max}$). Muscle wasting, impaired coordination, and decreased strength that results from an acute illness can also affect performance as well as increase risk of injury.

Studies have also shown that deconditioning of the cardiorespiratory, musculoskeletal, and metabolic systems can occur in athletes with less than 4 weeks off from training.[10] The effects are greatest, and occur most quickly, in the most highly trained athletes, sometimes beginning after only 4 to 5 days.[11] $Vo_{2max}$ can decline between 6% and 20% with deconditioning in highly trained athletes, affecting ventilatory efficiency and endurance.[12] Such decreases in exercise performance can last for 2 to 4 days beyond the complete resolution of an upper respiratory illness in athletes.[13] Research has shown that maintenance of low-level activity, when appropriate, can be used to fend off some of the physiologic changes associated with complete cessation of activity and should be considered in select cases.[12]

## Overtraining and Risk of Illness

The concept of overtraining cannot be ignored because it relates to risk of illness in athletes. Training philosophy centers on the idea of functional overreaching, whereby athletes push beyond normal limits in order to adapt to these higher loads and achieve gains in their sports. In order for this overreaching to benefit the athlete, adequate recovery needs to be factored into the equation. In situations in which there is not enough recovery, the athletes fail to improve and may see detrimental effects on their performance either in the form of nonfunctional overreaching or, in more extreme cases, overtraining syndrome. It is here that they are more susceptible to associated rates of increased illness and injury.

Experts have also acknowledged that the congested training and competition schedules of athletes, along with frequent travel, can lend themselves to both psychological and physiologic stress. These stressors can negatively affect health by increasing the risk of both overtraining syndrome as well as of contracting an acute illness.[14]

The International Olympic Committee convened an expert consensus group in 2015 that examined these constructs and concluded that the relationship between athletes' health and the loads placed on them should be seen as a well-being continuum along which load and recovery are mutual counteragents.[14,15] The amount of external and internal loads in the form of both sports-related and non–sports-related stressors places the athletes along a spectrum of health from homeostasis to acute fatigue, overreaching, overtraining syndromes and eventual immune changes, illness, and/or injury. With proper recognition of this disruption of the athlete's homeostasis, usually caused by having to stop for an illness or injury, rest can be initiated, resulting in recovery and return to homeostasis. If symptoms are ignored, this homeostasis remains out of balance and the athlete remains at risk for decreased performance and further illness/injury.

## RESPIRATORY INFECTIONS
### Upper Respiratory Tract Infection

Upper respiratory tract infections (URTIs) are the most common illnesses to affect both athletic and nonathletic populations alike. It has been reported that a typical adult is afflicted with a URTI 1 to 6 times per year.[9] Research indicates that more than 50% of acute illnesses reported during athletic competitions affect the upper respiratory tract.[14] Most URTIs are self-limited viral illnesses and their evaluation and treatment in athletes are typically the same as those of nonathletes. There are special considerations in athletes with regard to medication choices as well as appropriate timing of return to play.

### Cause
Most URTIs are in the category of the common cold and are caused by rhinoviruses. However, there are several other causative agents to consider because URTIs can also include the following illnesses: bronchitis, pharyngitis, sinusitis, influenza, infectious mononucleosis, and pertussis. Infections tend to occur in early autumn through early spring, with the greatest frequency occurring in the winter months. Athletes may be more at risk if they frequently travel for their sports, compete indoors, or have close contact with teammates and/or opponents. Rates of URTIs in athletes increase in the winter months, most likely because of crowding indoors, seasonal variations in pathogens, and physiologic changes that occur because of the cold.[16–18] In addition, athletes may be more susceptible to URTIs if they are under increased psychosocial stress, are undergoing a personal crisis, or are experiencing any type of sleep disturbance.[19,20]

### Diagnosis and treatment
URTIs are generally self-limited viral illnesses with the symptoms of rhinorrhea, sore throat, fatigue, nasal congestion, mildly increased temperature, and cough resolving within 7 to 10 days. The diagnosis is typically a clinical one that does not require testing, unless symptoms are prolonged or worsening and other pathogens are being considered.

Treatments often include over-the-counter medications, such as analgesics, antipyretics, and decongestants to aid in relief of symptoms, but these should be used judiciously (**Table 1**). Expectorants are generally considered safe and can help to thin mucus production. Antipyretics are also appropriate but should not be used solely to control a fever in order to allow participation. Caution should be used with first-generation antihistamines because they exert an anticholinergic effect that can result in fatigue, dehydration, and/or heat issues. Care should also be taken when using oral

**Table 1**
**Medications used with acute illnesses and potential risks in athletes**

| Medication | Potential Concerns in Athletes |
|---|---|
| Antibiotics: overall | Antibiotic-associated diarrhea<br>Theoretic risk of fatigue causing increased risk of injury |
| Fluoroquinolones | Tendinopathy<br>Tendon rupture<br>QTc prolongation<br>Photosensitivity |
| Macrolides | QTc prolongation |
| Tetracyclines/sulfonamides | Photosensitivity |
| Antihistamines:<br>  first generation | Anticholinergic effects = increased risk of dehydration and<br>  heat illness<br>Sedation = increased risk of injury |
| Antitussives | Fatigue = increased risk of injury |
| Antipyretics | Masks a fever |
| Beta-agonists | Tachycardia<br>May be banned in some sports |
| Oral decongestants | Increased risk of heat illness<br>May be banned in some sports |

decongestants in athletes because of risk of dehydration and hyperthermia, as well as restrictions on their use by certain sport governing bodies. Bronchodilators may be used short term to help with URTI-associated bronchospasm but are prohibited for use in some sports. Practitioners should always refer to the World Anti-Doping Agency (WADA) Web site for the most up-to-date list of prohibited substances if they are treating an Olympic sport athlete.[21]

### Prophylaxis
There is little in terms of preventive treatments against a URTI other than educating the athlete on maintenance of healthy lifestyle habits, such as consuming a nutritious diet, getting adequate sleep, not sharing water bottles, avoiding contact with infected individuals, and the practice of consistent hand washing and good coughing etiquette. Research is ongoing in terms of methods to monitor athletes for subclinical warning signs related to impending illness. At present, coaches and sports medicine staff should ensure adequate recovery is built into training programs, monitor for early signs of overload/overtraining such as fatigue and decreased performance, educate athletes on and encourage healthy habits/hygiene, and provide adequate time for administration of influenza vaccines and other needed immunizations related to travel (**Fig. 3**).

### Acute bronchitis

Acute bronchitis refers to a cough of infectious origin that lasts for more than 10 days but less than 3 weeks. A persistent cough can wreak havoc on an athlete's performance and training so there is often pressure on the medical team to find a solution.

### Cause
Viruses are the causative agent in acute bronchitis 90% of the time,[9,22] and include influenza A and B viruses, parainfluenza virus, respiratory syncytial virus, coronavirus, adenovirus, rhinovirus, and metapneumovirus. Bacterial causes include *Bordetella pertussis*, *Chlamydophila pneumoniae*, and *Mycoplasma pneumoniae*.

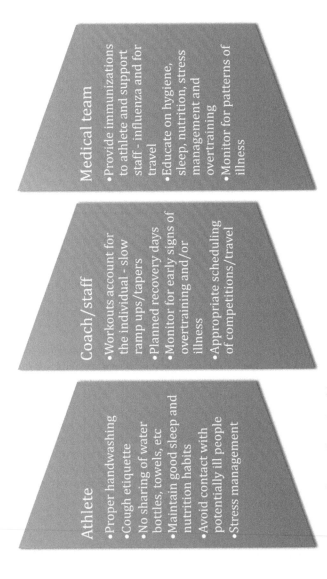

**Fig. 3.** Approach to prevention of acute illness in athletes.

### Diagnosis

Testing seldom needs to be performed to confirm the diagnosis because the diagnosis is made clinically from cough. Fever is unusual in most cases, but can be seen with influenza and pneumonia. Coughs of greater than 3 weeks should prompt investigation for pertussis, keeping in mind that a persistent cough can also be caused by asthma, gastroesophageal reflux, and postnasal drip.[23]

### Treatment

Treatment of acute bronchitis is directed at symptom relief in most cases. Evidence does not support the routine use of antibiotics.[23] Many athletes, and their coaches, expect antibiotics and it is important to educate them on the rationale for not doing so, which includes the avoidance of both antibiotic-associated diarrhea and antibiotic resistance.[23]

### Prophylaxis

As with most URTIs, there are no known preventive measures other than maintaining a healthy immune system and reducing the spread of infection, as described in **Fig. 3**.

### Pertussis

As previously mentioned, athletes with a cough lasting greater than 3 weeks warrant further evaluation. Although there are many potential causes of chronic cough, one highly infectious source that needs to be considered is pertussis.

### Cause

Pertussis is an infection caused by the bacterium *B pertussis*. It is typically spread person to person through aerosolized respiratory droplets. Infections in adults are usually mild and self-limited; nonetheless, a persistent cough can have a significant impact on an athlete's performance in most sports.

### Diagnosis

It can be difficult for clinicians to distinguish pertussis from other causes of chronic cough. Classic pertussis infection is described as having 3 phases of illness: catarrhal, paroxysmal, and convalescent. The catarrhal phase lasts 1 to 2 weeks and is characterized by a mild, intermittent cough, low-grade fevers, and coryza. In the paroxysmal phase, infected individuals experience a spasmodic cough, posttussive emesis, and an inspiratory whoop. This phase can range from 1 to 6 weeks in duration. The convalescent phase is when the symptoms begin to subside, typically over 7 to 10 days, but they can last for months.[24] The classic symptoms of posttussive emesis and whoop are rarely seen in clinical practice and, although their presence increases the specificity of pertussis, it is not enough to definitively diagnose pertussis.[25] Confirmatory testing for pertussis is via a nasopharyngeal swab, which can be sent for either culture or polymerase chain reaction (PCR). Results from culture have poor sensitivity and specificity and can take several days to obtain. PCR is costlier, but much quicker, with results available in 1 to 2 days. Because of such limitations, most suspected cases are treated based on patient presentation and ideally include known recent exposure to a confirmed index case.[25,26]

### Treatment

The earlier treatment of pertussis is started, the better. If the patient is able to start treatment in the first 1 to 2 weeks, before the onset of the coughing paroxysms, symptoms may be lessened. For this reason, clinicians should strongly consider treating based on clinical suspicion rather than waiting for confirmatory testing. *B pertussis* is considered contagious from the start of the catarrhal stage through the third week, after the onset of the paroxysmal phase, or until 5 days after the start of appropriate antibiotic treatment.[25] Antibiotic treatment that is started late does not alter the course of the illness and is unnecessary because pertussis is no longer considered infectious after ~21 days.

Macrolides are first-line agents for the treatment of pertussis, with trimethoprim-sulfamethoxazole being used when macrolides are contraindicated. Erythromycin was traditionally prescribed for 14 days, but, because of significant side effects and the lack of most people's ability to comply with a 4-times-per-day medication, azithromycin is more often chosen for treatment. In confirmed cases of pertussis, teammates and coaches should receive postexposure prophylaxis with the same macrolide treatment course. The American College of Chest Physicians (ACCP) states that once treatment of pertussis is initiated, the individual needs to be isolated for the first 5 days of antibiotic treatment. Therefore, athletes with pertussis need to be removed from contact with teammates and staff. Health care providers are mandated to report any confirmed cases.[25,27]

### Prophylaxis

There continue to be high rates of pertussis cases among teens and young adults despite improved immunization rates. These high rates are thought to be in part caused by a change from a live pertussis vaccine to an acellular version of the vaccine in the 1990s.[24] Based on these continued high rates of infection, the Advisory Council on Immunization Practices (ACIP) recommends a booster vaccine for adolescents and adults.[27,28] ACIP recommends a single Tdap dose for persons aged 11 to 18 years who have completed the primary series and for adults 19 to 64 years regardless of their last vaccine tetanus or diphtheria toxoid. In addition, pregnant women should receive a booster with each pregnancy, preferably between 27 and 36 weeks' gestation.[28] In the athletic setting, providers should be educating their athletes and staff about the importance of this vaccination.

### Influenza

Influenza is an extremely contagious viral respiratory illness that can spread quickly through an athletic program. The virus is easily transmitted via respiratory droplets, causing athletes to be at increased risk based on their close proximity to others during practice, competitions, and travel.

### Cause

Influenza subtypes A and B can be identified by rapid nasal swabs. Type B viruses only infect humans and mutate 2 to 3 times slower, resulting in a classically weaker strain that does not cause rapid spread. However, type A viruses are more virulent and can have many different animal hosts. The 2009 pandemic of H1N1 was credited with up to 403,000 hospitalizations, compared with the 200,000 seen in a typical flu season, and highlighted the challenges of not having an available vaccine against this influenza A strain.[29] Despite this, the concerted efforts of the US health care system to guide strong educational initiatives on hand washing, adherence to US Centers for Disease Control and Prevention (CDC) isolation guidelines, and the early reporting of symptoms helped to create awareness and contained many H1N1 outbreaks at the high school, collegiate, and professional sports levels.[30]

### Diagnosis

Classic influenza patients present with fever, dry cough, headache, and myalgias. Additional complaints can include a sore throat, rhinorrhea, and congestion. Diagnostic testing for influenza is typically not required in the care of the general population; however, confirming the diagnosis in athletes can be invaluable in prevention of a larger outbreak within an athletic program. Nasal washings or a pharyngeal swab should be obtained in an athlete presenting with the presumed index case during the influenza season. Once the index case is confirmed, any additional athletes with influenzalike symptoms can be presumed to also have influenza.

## Treatment

Otherwise healthy individuals infected with influenza usually have complete resolution with only symptomatic treatment.[31] Symptom improvement is seen between days 3 and 7, although cough and malaise can last days longer. Neuraminidase inhibitors (oseltamivir and zanamivir) can be used to treat influenza A and B, but in order to provide maximum effectiveness these medications need to be started within 48 hours of symptom onset.[32,33] Resistance to these medications is variable and changes over time.

Neuraminidase inhibitors are often considered for chemoprophylaxis in high-risk household contacts. In the 2009 H1N1 outbreak, athletes did not qualify for chemoprophylaxis based on CDC guidelines because they were not considered high-risk contacts, mainly because of a fear of antiviral shortages during the pandemic. In situations in which medication shortages are not a concern, clinicians should consider prophylaxis of an in-season sports team and their close contacts if a team member has confirmed influenza.

## Prophylaxis

Vaccination against influenza is the most important prevention strategy. ACIP recommends universal vaccination for those greater than 6 months of age.[34] Athletes and associated coaching staff members should be highly encouraged to obtain an influenza vaccine early because development of immunoprotection can take up to 5 weeks. In addition, vaccines should generally be scheduled in the off season, or as far away from important competitions as is possible.

## Respiratory Tract Infections and General Guidelines For Return To Play

Athletes with mild viral URTI can often continue to train and compete as tolerated provided that the severity and symptoms of the illness do not worsen with exercise.[19] Absolute contraindications to participation include fever, hypoxia, and dehydration. Practitioners should also take note of any athlete with unexplained sinus tachycardia because this is frequently the only sign of a viral-induced myocarditis after URTI.[35]

The so-called neck check has long been used as a guideline for when athletes may return to sport. If the symptoms are all above the neck, such as with rhinorrhea, sore throat, and nasal congestion, the athlete can attempt a return to activity. The athlete should start with a brief attempt at light exercise for 10 to 15 minutes, which can then be increased as tolerated assuming there is no worsening of the athlete's symptoms. If symptoms exist that are below the neck, such as fever, malaise, and gastrointestinal symptoms, the athlete should be kept from participation until symptoms have resolved.[20] Fever is a particularly concerning symptom that should not be masked with medication to allow participation. Athletes should be afebrile for at least 24 hours off any antipyretics before consideration for return to play.

When treating a bacterial infection such as sinusitis or pharyngitis, the athlete should be afebrile and on antibiotics for at least 24 hours before considering return to participation.[35] After this, a short trial of light activity can be undertaken and, if there is no effect on symptoms, then participation may be continued. However, if there is aggravation of significant symptoms, activity should be halted. Progression back to activity should be tailored to match the degree of illness that the athlete experienced. A good general rule of thumb is that for every day missed of training, the athlete should allow 2 to 3 days of graded return. The progression should also increase in small increments along the lines of 10% at a time, with frequency being increased first, followed by duration, and then intensity[35] (**Fig. 4**).

## GASTROINTESTINAL
### Traveler's Diarrhea

Traveler's diarrhea (TD) is an illness that affects up to 40% of travelers to resource-limited countries or regions. This risk includes athletes who travel to compete at the national or international level. Although TD is usually self-limited, the risk of secondary dehydration can adversely affect the athlete's ability to train and compete. Classically, TD presents with 3 or more unformed stools, nausea, vomiting, fever, abdominal cramping, or bloody stools. Most cases occur within the first 4 to 14 days of travel and last between 1 and 5 days.[36]

### Cause
Acute TD can be caused by 3 different infectious agents: bacteria, viruses, or parasites. About 90% of cases are bacterial, with most of those being caused by enterotoxic *Escherichia coli*.[37] Additional bacterial pathogens to consider include *Salmonella* species, *Shigella* species, *Vibrio* species, and *Campylobacter* species. Viruses cause up to 10% of TD cases, with Norovirus being the most frequent cause in adults. Parasitic organisms should also be considered in athletes with symptoms lasting longer than 7 days. Although only accounting for a small percentage of TD overall, common parasites include *Giardia lamblia*, *Cryptosporidium parvum*, and *Cyclospora cayetanensis*.[9]

### Diagnosis
The diagnosis of TD is typically made clinically and the pathogen is rarely isolated before symptoms resolve on their own. The diagnosis and approach to treatment used to be based on the number of unformed stools but now is based on a functional classification scheme (**Fig. 5**). Stool cultures should be obtained if the TD lasts greater than 7 days or the patient has fever or colitis symptoms (fever, tenesmus, urgency, cramping, or bloody diarrhea).[37,38]

### Treatment
The mainstay of treatment of TD is fluid replacement. Antibiotic therapy should be reserved for athletes that develop moderate to severe diarrhea, which is clinically classified by the International Society of Travel Medicine as distressing and interfering with planned activities; fever; or blood, pus, or mucus in the stool. Self-treatment with antibiotics for milder cases has been shown to increase microbial resistance.[39] In general, fluoroquinolones are avoided for treatment of TD in the athletic setting, because of potential effects on the musculoskeletal system, including the rare but worrisome risk of tendon rupture in athletes. Azithromycin has been shown to be as effective for TD as fluoroquinolones and is now the preferred agent.[40] Azithromycin is given as a 1000-mg single dose or as 500 mg daily for 3 days. In TD caused by *E coli*, rifaximin has been shown to be effective; however, it is not for use with any febrile diarrhea or dysentery.[41] If a parasitic cause is suspected, metronidazole 500 mg 3 times daily for 5 days is the preferred regimen. The use of antimotility agents such as loperamide and diphenoxylate has been considered controversial in the past, but it is now generally accepted as safe when taken with an antibiotic.[9] More conservative

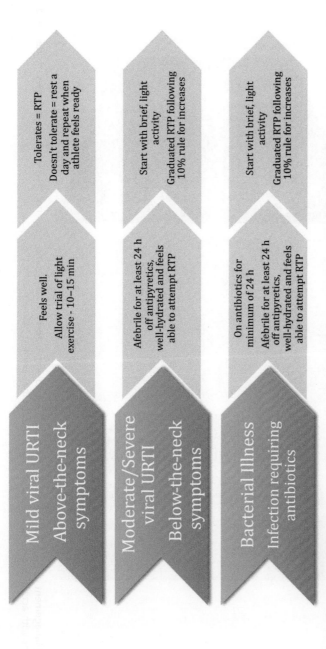

**Fig. 4.** General approach to return to play after acute illness in athletes. Specific infections may require additional considerations not listed here. RTP, return to play. (*Adapted from* Jaworski CA, Pyne DB. Upper respiratory tract infections: Considerations in adolescent and adult athletes. UpToDate. Accessed November 26, 2018.)

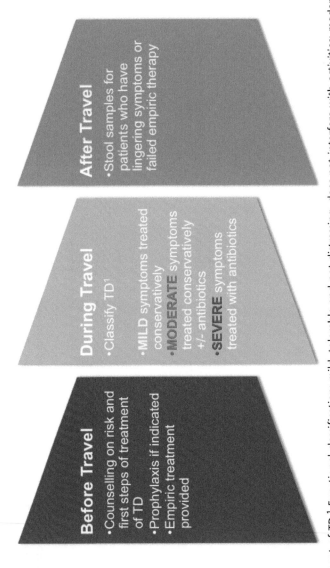

**Before Travel**
- Counselling on risk and first steps of treatment of TD
- Prophylaxis if indicated
- Empiric treatment provided

**During Travel**
- Classify TD[1]
- **MILD** symptoms treated conservatively
- **MODERATE** symptoms treated conservatively +/- antibiotics
- **SEVERE** symptoms treated with antibiotics

**After Travel**
- Stool samples for patients who have lingering symptoms or failed empiric therapy

**Fig. 5.** Management of TD.[1] Functional classification: mild, tolerable and not distressing, does not interfere with activities; moderate, distressing or interferes with activities; severe, incapacitating symptoms that prevent planned activities.

recommendations for use in athletes suggest reserving it for use only preceding a competition or during a long trip.[42] A summary of the recommendations for TD treatment can be found in **Table 2**.

### Prophylaxis and special considerations

Although antibiotics can be used effectively as prophylaxis in TD, they should not be used routinely. Antibiotic prophylaxis should be reserved for athletes that have underlying health conditions, such as severe inflammatory bowel disease, advanced human immunodeficiency virus, or complicated organ transplant, that would put them at high risk of morbidity if they developed TD. If prophylaxis is needed for an athlete, rifaximin is the antibiotic currently recommended at either 200 mg daily, twice daily, or 3 times daily because of a much lower side effect profile than the fluoroquinolones.[43] Before travel to high-risk regions, athletes should be educated on prudent selection of food and drinks. Selecting only bottled water or carbonated canned drinks, both consumed from the bottle with a straw rather than from a glass, as well as only eating fully cooked hot food and fruit that is peeled by the eater can minimize risk. Avoidance of buffets, condiments, ice, and food provided on international return flights are additional measures that should be taken while athletes are traveling. Of course, proper handwashing and avoidance of sharing utensils or glassware are also necessary to minimize risk.

### Return to play

The return-to-play plan can be initiated once an athlete is afebrile, rehydrated, and back to tolerating solid foods with no residual gastrointestinal symptoms. Care should be taken to progress slowly through conditioning and then more intense training to allow for any possible deconditioning that occurred, following the same guidelines as outlined for URTIs.

## GENITOURINARY
### Urinary Tract Infections

Urinary tract infection (UTI) is a frequently seen condition that affects women much more often than men. One-third of all women experience at least 1 UTI before the age of 24 years, and is therefore a common reason for female high school and college athletes to seek medical attention.[44]

**Table 2**
**Approved treatment regimens for traveler's diarrhea**

| Agent | Dose (mg) | Duration | Comment |
|---|---|---|---|
| Azithromycin | 1000 once<br>500 daily | Single dose<br>3 d | Preferred for dysentery, febrile diarrheas, south east Asia travelers, pregnant women |
| Levofloxacin | 500 daily | Single or 3 d | FQ are associated with tendon rupture |
| Ciprofloxacin | 750 once<br>500 twice daily | Single dose | and _Clostridium difficile_ |
| Ofloxacin | 400 daily | 3 d | |
| Rifaximin | 200 3 times daily | 3 d | Not used with dysentery or febrile diarrhea |
| Metronidazole | 500 3 times daily | 5 d | When parasitic infection is suspected |

_Abbreviation:_ FQ, fluoroquinolone.

### Cause

*E coli* is the most common cause of UTI in both men and women and accounts for 75% to 95% of cases in women. Less common pathogens include other Entero-bacteriaceae, such as *Klebsiella pneumoniae* and *Proteus mirabilis*. In athletes with recent hospitalizations or antimicrobial use, organisms such as *Pseudomonas*, entero-cocci, and staphylococci should be considered as well.[45]

### Diagnosis

The diagnosis of UTI can often be accomplished by patient history alone. Female ath-letes presenting with symptoms of dysuria and frequency have a 90% probability of UTI and may be treated empirically without further testing. Cystitis in male athletes and atypical/vague symptoms in either gender warrant laboratory testing with urinal-ysis and urine culture to confirm the diagnosis.[46]

### Treatment

First-line antimicrobial agents include trimethoprim-sulfamethoxazole (TMP-SMX) and nitrofurantoin. Choice of agent often comes down to factors such as patient allergies, tolerance of the medication, or local resistance patterns. Of note, TMP-SMX has seen a large increase in the rate of resistance in the past 30 years.[47] Resistance rates vary based on geography, but TMP-SMX is still considered a first-line choice when rates are less than 20%.[47] Women with uncomplicated infection are treated with a 3-day course of antibiotics.[48,49] Men with cystitis require both a urinalysis and urine culture for their work-up, along with a 7-day course of therapy.[50]

### Prophylaxis

Several studies have suggested that drinking cranberry juice may decrease the inci-dence of UTIs. A recent meta-analysis from 2017 found that cranberry reduced the risk for UTI by 26% in otherwise healthy nonpregnant women with a history of UTIs. Studies reviewed were small in sample size, most with fewer than 300 participants. A larger, higher-quality study is needed for further investigation.[51]

### Return to play

Athletes should be restricted from participation until they are afebrile, hydration is restored, and urinary symptoms have resolved. Uncomplicated UTI in female athletes should not significantly hamper training if treatment is started at the onset of symp-toms. More serious cases require the athletes to have completed their antibiotic treat-ment and may warrant a graduated return to participation to account for possible deconditioning.

## Sexually transmitted infections

Sexually transmitted infections continue to plague society, with individuals 15 to 24 years old accounting for half of all new infections. Because many athletes are within this age range, educational initiatives are paramount in preventing spread of disease.[52]

### Cause

In 2017, the CDC reported that nearly 2.3 million cases of chlamydia, gonorrhea, and syphilis were diagnosed in the United States, marking the fourth consecutive year of sharp increases in these diseases.[52] Regardless, human papillomavirus (HPV) is still the most common sexually transmitted disease despite vaccine availability.

*Diagnosis*

Symptomatic athletes or those exposed to sexually transmitted diseases should be tested. For routine health maintenance, the United States Preventive Services Task Force (USPSTF) recommends screening for sexually transmitted diseases in asymptomatic individuals according to **Table 3**. All sexually active women up to the age of 24 years, or older women that are at increased risk, should be screened for chlamydia and gonorrhea. However, for asymptomatic men, there is insufficient evidence to screen. Syphilis is tested for in any individual deemed to be at increased risk, including suspected exposure, decreased immune system, or pregnancy. HPV is only screened for in women between the ages of 30 and 65 years in the form of cotesting during pap smears. Before the age of 30 years, most women can clear HPV infections, therefore it is not recommended to routinely test.[53]

*Treatment*

The CDC recommendations for treatments for sexually transmitted diseases are listed in **Table 4**. Treatment of gonorrhea now includes dual-antibiotic therapy with the addition of azithromycin because of emerging antibiotic resistance to ceftriaxone alone. In the treatment of syphilis, the only approved therapy is penicillin by intramuscular injection. For individuals allergic to penicillin, the recommendation is to undergo desensitization because there is no alternative medication. HPV is managed with lesion destruction, including cryotherapy and topical erosive agents.[53]

*Prophylaxis*

The USPSTF recommends behavioral counseling for all sexually active adolescents and adults with safe sex practices as a preventive measure for sexually transmitted diseases. In addition, there is currently a vaccine available for both men and women to protect against HPV. Gardasil is recommended starting at age 9 years, and recent change in US Food and Drug Administration regulations allow it to be administered up to age 45 years. Although the vaccine does not protect against all strains of the HPV virus, it offers protection against several of the high-risk strains.[52]

*Return to Play*

Return-to-play guidelines are based on the cause and severity of infection. Uncomplicated infections, such as chlamydial or gonorrheal urethritis/cervicitis/rectal disease, rarely warrant exclusion from participation. Any complications, such as epididymitis, pelvic inflammatory disease, or disseminated gonococcal disease, should result in the athlete being held from competition until all symptoms have

**Table 3**
**United States Preventive Services Task Force recommendations for screening for sexually transmitted diseases**

| STD | USPSTF Recommendations for Screening | |
| --- | --- | --- |
| | **Women** | **Men** |
| Chlamydia | Up to age 24 y if sexually active, or older if increased risk | Insufficient evidence |
| Gonorrhea | Up to age 24 y if sexually active, or older if increased risk | Insufficient evidence |
| Syphilis | Any at increased risk for infection | Any at increased risk for infection |
| HPV | Every 5 y in ages 30–60 y with pap smear | Not indicated |

*Abbreviation:* STD, sexually transmitted disease.

**Table 4**
**United States Centers for Disease Control and Prevention recommended treatment regimens for sexually transmitted disease**

| STD | Recommended Treatment Regimen |
| --- | --- |
| Chlamydia | Azithromycin 1 g once, or |
| | Doxycycline 100 mg twice daily for 7 d |
| Gonorrhea | Ceftriaxone 250 mg intramuscularly, pus |
| | Azithromycin 1 g once or doxycycline 100 mg twice daily for 7 d |
| Syphilis | |
|   Primary and secondary | Benzathine penicillin G 2.4 million units IM |
|   Tertiary | Benzathine penicillin G 7.2 million units IM given over 3 doses each 1 wk apart |
| HPV | Lesion destruction |

*Abbreviation:* IM, intramuscular.

resolved. Once symptoms are resolved, the athlete can partake in a graduated return-to-play progression.[52]

## SUMMARY

Understanding the impact that an acute illness can impart on an athlete's training and performance, as well as the caveats in creating a treatment and return-to-play plan, is essential when providing care to athletes. The general principles of returning an athlete to training should center on ensuring a gradual progression that takes into account any deconditioning that occurred over the course of the illness. Staying up to date on the best treatment approaches as well as monitoring for any signs or symptoms of overtraining helps to keep athletes in the game.

## REFERENCES

1. Gleeson M. Immune function in sport and exercise. J Appl Physiol 2007;103: 693–9.
2. Nieman DC. Exercise, infection and immunity. Int J Sports Med 1994;15:S131–41.
3. Campbell JP, Turner JE. Debunking the myth of exercise-induced immune suppression: Redefining the impact of exercise on immunological health across the lifespan. Front Immunol 2018;9:648.
4. Ekblom B, Ekblom O, Malm C. Infectious episodes before and after a marathon race. Scand J Med Sci Sports 2006;16:287.
5. Hellard P, Avalos M, Guimaraes F, et al. Training-related risk of common illnesses in elite swimmers over a 4-year period. Med Sci Sports Exerc 2015;47:698–707.
6. Veugelers KR, Young WB, Fahrner B, et al. Different methods of training load quantification and their relationship to injury and illness in elite Australian football. J Sci Med Sport 2016;19:24–8.
7. Mårtensson S, Nordebo K, Malm C. High training volumes are associated with a low number of self-reported sick days in elite endurance athletes. J Sports Sci Med 2014;13:929–33.
8. Malm C. Susceptibility to infections in elite athletes: the S-curve. Scand J Med Sci Sports 2006;16:4–6.

9. Jaworski CA, Donahue B, Kluetz J. Infectious disease. Clin Sports Med 2011; 30:575.

10. Mujika I, Padilla S. Detraining: loss of training-induced physiological and performance adaptations. Part I. Sports Med 2000;30:79–87.

11. Lorenc TM, Kernan MT. Lower respiratory infections and potential complications in athletes. Curr Sports Med Rep 2006;5(2):80–6.

12. Mujika I, Padilla S. Detraining: loss of training-induced physiological and performance adaptations. Part II. Sports Med 2000;30:145–54.

13. Schwellnus MP, Schwellnus MP, Jeans A, et al. Exercise and infections. In: Schwellnus MP, editor. The Olympic textbook of medicine in sport. Oxford: Wiley-Blackwell; 2008. p. 344–64.

14. Schwellnus M, Soligard T, Alonso J-M, et al. How much is too much? (Part 2) International Olympic Committee consensus statement on load in sport and risk of illness. Br J Sports Med 2016;50:1043–52.

15. Fry RW, Morton AR, Keast D. Overtraining in athletes. An update. Sports Med 1991;12:32–65.

16. Orhant E, Carling C, Cox A. A three-year prospective study of illness in professional soccer players. Res Sports Med 2010;18(3):199–204.

17. Mountjoy M, Junge A, Alonso JM, et al. Sports injuries and illnesses in the 2009 FINA World Championships (Aquatics). Br J Sports Med 2010;44(7):522–7.

18. Castellani JW, Brenner IK, Rhind SG. Cold exposure: human immune responses and intracellular cytokine expression. Med Sci Sports Exerc 2002;34:2013–20.

19. Metz JP. Upper respiratory tract infections: who plays, who sits? Curr Sports Med Rep 2003;2:84–90.

20. Eichner ER. Infection, immunity, and exercise: what to tell your patients. Physician Sports Med 1993;21:125.

21. WADA prohibited list. Available at: http://www.wada-ama.org/en/what-we-do/the-prohibited-list. Accessed November 26, 2018.

22. Braman SS. Chronic cough due to acute bronchitis: ACCP evidence-based clinical practice guidelines. Chest 2006;129(1 suppl):955–1035.

23. Smoot MK, Hosey RG. Pulmonary infections in the athlete. Curr Sports Med Rep 2009;8(2):71–5.

24. Centers for Disease Control and Prevention. Recommended antimicrobial agents for the treatment and postexposure prophylaxis of pertussis. Available at: https://www.cdc.gov/mmwr/preview/mmwrhtml/rr5414a1.htm. Accessed November 26, 2018.

25. Centers for Disease Control and Prevention. Pertussis treatment. Available at: https://www.cdc.gov/pertussis/clinical/treatment.html. Accessed November 26, 2018.

26. Cornia PB, Hersh AL, Lipshy BA, et al. Does this coughing adolescent or adult patient have pertussis? JAMA 2010;304:890–6.

27. Liang JL, Tiwari T, Moro P, et al. Prevention of pertussis, tetanus, and diphtheria with vaccines in the United States: recommendations of the Advisory Committee on Immunization Practices (ACIP). MMWR Recomm Rep 2018;67(No. RR-2):1–44.

28. Centers for Disease Control and Prevention. Pertussis: summary of vaccine recommendations. Available at: http://www.cdc.gov/vaccines/vpd-vac/pertussis/recs-summary.htm. Accessed November 26, 2018.

29. Centers for Disease Control and Prevention. Updated CDC estimates of 2009 H1N1 influenza cases, hospitalizations and deaths in the United States, April

2009-April 10, 2010. Available at: http://www.cdc.gov/h1n1flu/estimates_2009_h1n1.htm. Accessed December 14, 2010.

30. Dawood FS, Jain S, Finelli L, et al, Novel Swine-Origin Influenza A (H1N1) Virus Investigation Team. Emergence of a novel swine-origin influenza A (H1N1) virus in humans. N Engl J Med 2009;360:2605–15.

31. Harper SA, Bradley JS, Englund JA, et al. Seasonal influenza in adults and children-diagnosis, treatment, chemoprophylaxis, and institutional outbreak management: clinical practice guidelines of the Infectious Diseases Society of America. Clin Infect Dis 2009;48:1003–32.

32. Jefferson T, Jones M, Doshi P, et al. Neuraminidase inhibitors for preventing and treating influenza in healthy adults: systemic review and meta-analysis. BMJ 2009;339:b5106.

33. Treanor JJ, Hayden FG, Vrooman PS, et al. US Oral Neuraminidase Study Group. Efficacy and safety of the oral neuraminidase inhibitor oseltamivir in treating acute influenza: a randomized controlled trial. JAMA 2000;283:1016–24.

34. Advisory Committee on Immunization Practices. Influenza ACIP vaccine recommendations. Available at: https://www.cdc.gov/vaccines/hcp/acip-recs/vacc-specific/flu.html. Accessed November 26, 2018.

35. Jaworski CA, Pyne DB. Upper respiratory tract infections: considerations in adolescent and adult athletes. UpToDate. Available at: https://www.uptodate.com/contents/upper-respiratory-tract-infections-considerations-in-adolescent-and-adult-athletes. Accessed November 26, 2018.

36. Hill DR. Occurrence and self-treatment of diarrhea in a large cohort of Americans traveling to developing countries. Am J Trop Med Hyg 2000;62:585–9.

37. DuPont HL, Ericsson CD. Prevention and treatment of traveler's' diarrhea. N Engl J Med 1993;328:1821–7.

38. Goodgame R. Emerging causes of traveler's diarrhea: Cryptosporidium, Cyclospora, Isospora, and Microsporidia. Curr Infect Dis Rep 2003;5:66–73.

39. Kantele A, Laaveri T, Mero S, et al. Antimicrobials increase traveler's risk of colonization by extended-spectrum betalactamase-producing Enterobacteriaceae. Clin Infect Dis 2015;60(6):837.

40. Adachi JA, Ericsson CD, Jiang ZD, et al. Azithromycin found to be comparable to levofloxacin for the treatment of US travelers with acute diarrhea acquired in Mexico. Clin Infect Dis 2003;37:1165–71.

41. Adachi JA, DuPont HL. Rifaximin: a novel nonabsorbed refamycin for gastrointestinal disorders. Clin Infect Dis 2006;42:541–7.

42. Murphy GS, Bodhidatta L, Echeverria P, et al. Ciprofloxacin and loperamide in the treatment of bacillary dysentery. Ann Intern Med 1993;118:582–6.

43. Riddle MS, Connor BA, Beeching NJ, et al. Guidelines for the prevention and treatment of traveler's' diarrhea: a graded expert panel report. J Travel Med 2017;24:S57.

44. Dielubanza EJ, Schaeffer AJ. Urinary tract infections in women. Med Clin North Am 2011;95:27–41.

45. Echols RM, Tosiello RL, Haverstock, et al. Demographic, clinical, and treatment parameters influencing the outcome of acute cystitis. Clin Infect Dis 1999;29(1):113.

46. Bent S, Nallamothu BK, Simel DL, et al. Does this woman have an acute uncomplicated urinary tract infection? JAMA 2002;287(20):2701.

47. Zhanel GG, Hisanaga TL, Laing NM, et al. Antibiotic resistance in outpatient urinary isolates: final results from the North American urinary tract infection collaborative alliance (NAUTICA). Int J Antimicrob Agents 2006;27:468–75.

48. Wagenlehner FM, Weidner W, Naber KG. An update on uncomplicated urinary tract infections in women. Curr Opin Urol 2009;19:268–74.
49. Milo G, Katchman E, Paul M, et al. Duration of antibacterial treatment for uncomplicated urinary tract infections in women. Cochrane Database Syst Rev 2005;(2):CD004682.
50. Raynor MC, Carson CC III. Urinary infections in men. Med Clin North Am 2011;95: 43–54.
51. Fu Z, Liska D, Talon D, et al. Cranberry reduces the risk of urinary tract infection recurrence in otherwise healthy women: a systematic review and meta-analysis. J Nutr 2017;147(12):2282–8.
52. Centers for Disease Control and Prevention. New CDC analysis shows step and sustained increases in STDs in recent years. 2018. Available at: https://www.cdc.gov/nchhstp/newsroom/2018/press-release-2018-std-prevention-conference.html. Accessed November 26, 2018.
53. United States Preventive Services Task Force. Available at: https://www.uspreventiveservicestaskforce.org/BrowseRec/Index/browse-recommendations. Accessed November 26, 2018.

# Sports Dermatology
## Skin Disease in Athletes

Patrick C. Carr, MD, Thomas G. Cropley, MD*

### KEYWORDS

- Skin disorders in athletes • Athletic skin infections • Mechanical skin disease
- Contact dermatitis

### KEY POINTS

- Mechanically induced skin diseases are most common in athletes and may affect training and performance.
- Inflammatory conditions such as contact dermatitis tend to be sport specific; thus management requires knowledge of equipment and environment.
- Skin infections are a common issue in sports dermatology, due to close contact with other athletes, poor cleaning of equipment, environment, and trauma.

## INTRODUCTION

There are numerous skin disorders that occur in athletes, which include infections, mechanical injury, and inflammatory skin diseases such as dermatitis, urticaria, and others. This article discusses some of the most common athletic skin diseases.

## MECHANICALLY INDUCED DERMATOLOGIC DISEASE

Athletic activities inherently involve trauma of various forms to the skin, regardless of whether or not the sport is considered a "contact" sport. Repetitive trauma to the skin is known to cause alteration in skin structure and can develop many cutaneous manifestations as a result. The most common example of this would include simple calluses due to repetitive trauma to specific areas.[1]

Some sports are more prone to frictional changes due to repeated motions such as running, racket sports, baseball, golf, or any sport involving repetitive equipment contact. Here, the authors review some of the common dermatologic conditions that are encountered frequently in a university athletic setting or by a primary care physician.

Department of Dermatology, University of Virginia, PO Box 800718, Charlottesville, VA 22908, USA
* Corresponding author.
E-mail address: Tgc3ge@virginia.edu

Clin Sports Med 38 (2019) 597–618
https://doi.org/10.1016/j.csm.2019.06.001
0278-5919/19/© 2019 Elsevier Inc. All rights reserved.

sportsmed.theclinics.com

### Friction Blister

- Diagnosis and presentation[2–7]
  - A vesicle or bulla that forms in an area of repetitive high frictional stress normally with some associated pain and tenderness (**Fig. 1**). It is caused by mechanical separation of the epidermal cells at the level of the stratum spinosum in areas of skin exposed to high lateral frictional forces. The blister is normally filled with clear fluid that is similar in composition to plasma; however, it can be hemorrhagic with the most common sites located on the tips of the toes, the balls of the feet, and the posterior heel. There is a higher incidence with increased heat, moisture, and sudden increase in new activities. Physical examination and history of friction in the area usually provides a clear clinical diagnosis. In the absence of high frictional forces to the area, it is important to thoroughly evaluate the area for another cause. A case has been reported of a patient who developed a hemorrhagic blister overlying a melanoma.[8]
- Treatment
  - If painful, the bulla or vesicle can be incised and drained with a sterile #11 blade and dressed with antiseptic, petroleum jelly, and clean bandage.
- Prevention
  - Acrylic socks have been shown to be more effective at the prevention of blisters than cotton socks.[3]

### Callus

- Diagnosis and presentation[4,7,9–11]
  - These present as areas of thickened, hyperkeratotic papules or plaques (**Fig. 2**). They are normally painless in comparison to corns. It is a protective response of the skin with hyperkeratinization and thickening of the stratum corneum.[7] It occurs most often in areas of high friction such as the feet of runners or hands of batters.[7,12]
- Treatment
  - No treatment is necessary and often calluses can help prevent the development of blisters.
  - If treatment is desired
    - Keratolytic creams: urea, salicylic acid.
    - Simple debridement.
- Prevention
  - Wearing gloves or other protective layers.

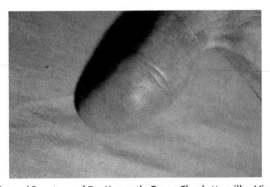

**Fig. 1.** Friction blister. (*Courtesy of* Dr. Kenneth Greer Charlottesville, Virginia.)

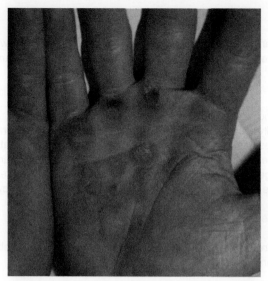

**Fig. 2.** Calluses. (*Courtesy of* Dr. Kenneth Greer Charlottesville, Virginia.)

## Corn

- Diagnosis and presentation[2,4,7,9–11]
  - Corns are punctate papules with a deep hyperkeratotic core that normally occur over a bony prominence (**Fig. 3**). Often there is associated tenderness with palpation to the lesion. They are commonly misdiagnosed as warts. The most common locations are the plantar surface of the great toes and distal head of the metatarsals.
- Treatment
  - Short-term treatment is the repeated removal of the overlying hyperkeratotic core with a #15 blade after overnight application of salicylic acid. Offloading pads found at most drug stores also help prevent lesions and permit healing over time.
- Prevention
  - Proper fitting footwear and wearing offloading corn pads can be helpful.
- Differential
  - Callus
    - Unlike corns, a callus does not have central hyperkeratotic core.[13]

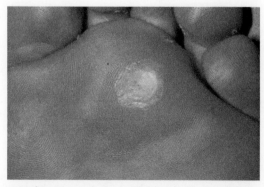

**Fig. 3.** Corn. (*Courtesy of* Dr. Kenneth Greer Charlottesville, Virginia.)

○ Wart
■ Callus and corns do not have capillary thrombi, whereas warts do.[13]
■ Callus retains skin line markings, which are lost in warts and can be lost in corns.[10]

### Talon Noir

- Diagnosis and presentation[2,5,10]
  ○ It is normally seen in adolescents or young adults. Talon noir (literally, "black heel") usually presents as horizontally arranged dark hyperpigmentation at the upper edge of the heel (**Fig. 4**). It occurs secondary to intracorneal and subepidermal hemorrhage from sports that produce shearing/pinching stress at the upper edge of the calcaneal fat pad. It can be confused with melanocytic lesions.
- Treatment
  ○ No treatment is needed.
- Prevention
  ○ Slowly increase new sporting activities and start wearing a felt heel pad in the area if prone to lesions.
- Differential
  ○ Melanocytic neoplasms, including melanoma. Biopsy or refer to dermatology if there is doubt.

### Subungual Hematoma

- Diagnosis and presentation[1,2,6,14–17]
  ○ This is defined as a small area of hemorrhage underneath the nail bed (**Fig. 5**). If located on a toe, it is called "tennis toe," "joggers toe," "skiers toe," or "hikers toe." Usually, clinical examination can adequately diagnose hemorrhage with magnification and red hue of the lesion. This condition is caused by repetitive contact of the toe anteriorly against the shoe or frequent dorsiflexion of the toes in a shoe with a restricted toe box. If concerned for melanoma, referral to dermatology for biopsy is appropriate.
- Treatment
  ○ Rest and foot soaking are usually adequate; however, drainage of blood under the nail can result in immediate pain relief. If pain is severe consider imaging with radiograph to evaluate for underlying fracture.
  ○ See Siobhan Statuta and Kelli Pugh's article, "Athletic Training Room Procedures and Use of Therapeutic Modalities," in this issue, Procedures and Modalities, for management.

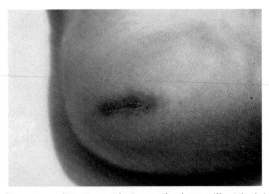

**Fig. 4.** Talon noir. (*Courtesy of* Dr. Kenneth Greer Charlottesville, Virginia.)

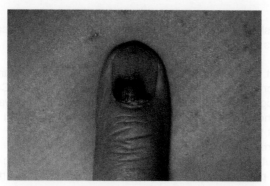

**Fig. 5.** Subungual hematoma. (*Courtesy of* Dr. Kenneth Greer Charlottesville, Virginia.)

- Prevention
  - Good fitting footwear, trimming toenails, and using a toe pad in the affected area can be helpful.

### Piezogenic Papules (Cutaneous Hernia)

- Diagnosis and presentation[15,17]
  - These are skin-colored papules and nodules on lateral surface of feet that result due to subdermal fat herniation from prolonged standing or exercise (**Fig. 6**). They are often accentuated when the athlete bears weight or stands and can disappear with foot elevation. It occurs most commonly in long-distance runners.[17]
- Prevention
  - Overweight individuals with rapid starting and stopping motions are at higher risk. Decreasing activity level and weight loss is beneficial.
- Treatment
  - No treatment is necessary.

### Turf Toe

- Diagnosis and presentation[2,14,18–20]
  - A painful, red, and swollen great toe that occurs because of underlying tendonitis of the flexor and extensor tendons within the great toe. This is most commonly seen in athletes who play on turf fields during sports that involve rapid start-stop maneuvers such as football or soccer.

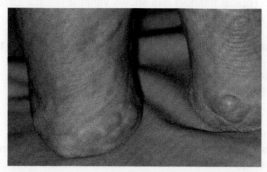

**Fig. 6.** Piezogenic papules. (*Courtesy of* Dr. Kenneth Greer Charlottesville, Virginia.)

- Prevention
  - Wearing shoes with adequate cushion and compression can help prevent symptoms if turf fields cannot be avoided.
- Treatment
  - Icing, rest, nonsteroidal antiinflammatory drugs, and avoidance of causative activity for 2 to 3 weeks usually resolves the symptoms. Consider imaging with radiograph initially to rule out fracture, then MRI for evaluation if symptoms do not resolve after weeks with a negative radiograph or extreme pain is present that does not fit a diagnosis.
- Differential diagnosis
  - Acute gouty arthritis or acute paronychia should also be considered; however, history of predisposing activities to turf toe indicates the diagnosis.

## Jogger's Nipples

- Diagnosis and presentation[1,5,10,18,19]
  - Presents early as painful eroded dermatitis of the nipples that is due to repetitive friction of the athlete's shirt on protruding joggers' nipples. It mainly occurs in men wearing hard fabrics such as polyesters for long periods of time while running or in women who do not wear a bra.
- Treatment
  - The main goal is prevention of further dermatitis to allow healing. If suspected superficial infection is present, topical mupirocin ointment can be beneficial. Otherwise, petroleum jelly applied regularly throughout the day will expedite healing.
- Prevention
  - Wearing a sports bra in women or for men, forgoing a shirt altogether.
  - Protective bandage over the nipples.
  - Petroleum jelly before runs.

## Striae Distensae

- Diagnosis and presentation[2,7,17,18]
  - Striae distensae presents as pink linear atrophic plaques over areas of the skin with underlying hypertrophy of muscle or repetitive stretching (**Fig. 7**) and is caused by rupture of elastic fibers in the reticular dermis. It most commonly occurs over the anterior shoulders, lower back, and thighs in athletes; however, it can present in any location that has undergone underlying rapid growth.
- Treatment
  - Treatment is often difficult and is mainly focused on the cosmetic aspects of the lesion. Topical tretinoin has shown variable results. Laser therapies can be helpful as well as medical tattooing.
- Prevention
  - Avoiding anabolic steroids, which have been associated with the development of striae distensae.
  - Slow increase in weightlifting activities.
  - Avoiding rapid weight gain.

## Athletes Nodule

- Diagnosis and presentation[10,21]
  - Nodules normally present as asymptomatic and flesh colored in areas that experience high friction or repetitive trauma such as the feet, hands, or knees (**Fig. 8**). These are considered a distinct form of a callus. They often occur

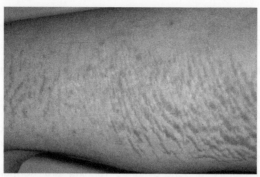

**Fig. 7.** Striae distensae. (*Courtesy of* Dr. Kenneth Greer Charlottesville, Virginia.)

secondary to the equipment used by the athlete, such as underpads for football players or in "hot spots" of shoes.
- Treatment
  - None required and are often desirable for protection during athletic activity.
  - If painful or symptomatic, surgical or laser removal is possible.
  - Application of urea cream or salicylic acid to soften and remove the keratinization can be helpful.
  - Intralesional steroids have also been used in the past but usually are not necessary.
- Prevention
  - Depending on the causative factor, avoiding the athletic activity or obtaining better fitting equipment may be helpful. The goal is to remove the repetitive trauma to the affected area.

### Golfers Nails

- Diagnosis and presentation[2,18,22]
  - Golfers nails present as linear dark streaks on a golfer's fingernail secondary to splinter hemorrhages within the nail. It occurs secondary to gripping the shaft of the club too tightly, which causes increased intravascular pressure and results in hemorrhage of the nail plate vasculature. Diagnosis normally can be made with physical examination and appreciation of red hue (blood) under the nail with magnification.

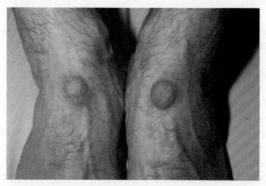

**Fig. 8.** Athlete nodules. (*Courtesy of* Dr. Kenneth Greer Charlottesville, Virginia.)

- Treatment
  - No treatment is required, and condition normally resolves spontaneously with correction of grip.
- Prevention
  - Education regarding proper grip with decreased grip tension.

### Runners Rump

- Diagnosis and presentation[2,6,15,18]
  - The rump presents with hyperpigmentation on the superior aspect of the gluteal cleft in long-distance runners due to small underlying ecchymosis. It is thought to occur from friction in long-distances runners. Physical examination and a history of long-distance running are normally adequate for diagnosis.
- Treatment
  - Usually asymptomatic and no treatment is required.
- Prevention
  - Altering the clothing choice to softer materials.
  - Topical lubricants applied to the area before, during, and after the run can be effective.

### Rowers Rump

- Diagnosis and presentation[1,2,14]
  - This presents as areas of well-demarcated, lichenified plaques of the buttocks, similar to lichen simplex chronicus. It normally occurs in areas that make contact with an unpadded seat of a rower. Cyclists develop identical lesions ("saddle sores"). The diagnosis is made with history and physical examination.
- Treatment
  - Intralesional or topical high potency steroid for lichenified areas to decrease lichenification and alleviate associated pruritus.
- Prevention
  - A padded seat or shorts with added cushion in the rear portion can be helpful.

### Swimmer's Shoulder

- Diagnosis and presentation[2,18,19,23]
  - This presents as a plaque that develops secondary to a swimmer's beard repetitively rubbing against his shoulder and is similar in pathogenesis to lichen simplex chronicus. Skin hypertrophy and irritation occurs from this repeated trauma. History and physical examination can lead to the correct diagnosis.
- Treatment
  - Shaving before swimming will allow the lesion to resolve in weeks to months. Topical steroids can be helpful if the lesion is pruritic.
- Prevention
  - Shaving daily can prevent the reoccurrence of the lesion.

### Erythema Ab Igne

- Diagnosis and presentation[10,24,25]
  - It presents as an erythematous or hyperpigmented reticulate patch often occurring on the back yet can appear anywhere (**Fig. 9**). This is a cutaneous reaction that results from chronic, repeated exposure to a heat source such as a heating pad. History and physical examination identifying the characteristic appearance of the rash is adequate for diagnosis.[10]

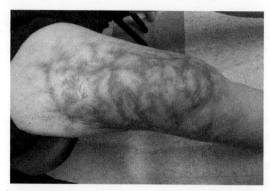

**Fig. 9.** Erythema ab igne. (*Courtesy of* Dr. Barrett Zlotoff Charlottesville, Virginia.)

- Treatment
  - Avoiding heat sources to the area will cause spontaneous resolution.
- Prevention
  - Recognition of the lesion and avoiding heat to the area after it develops.
- Important consideration
  - A small chance of developing into skin cancer has been noted; therefore, it is important to diagnose, discontinue further heat to the area, and monitor closely for resolution.

## Inflammatory conditions

Multiple forms of inflammatory dermatitis of different causes can occur in the athletic setting. Contact dermatitis is very common. Most studies have involved occupational dermatitis in industrialized nations. This incidence has been found to be as high as 30%, with 90% of that number due to irritant or allergic contact dermatitis (ACD).[26] It is often difficult to differentiate the cause of contact dermatitis from irritant or allergic. Irritant is more common than contact, with some estimations attributing 80% to irritant contact dermatitis (ICD) versus only 20% to allergic. Timing can be helpful for differentiating the type of contact dermatitis. Generally, ACD requires a previous exposure and develops hours to days after reexposure to that same substance. ACD is a CD4+, T-cell–mediated, delayed hypersensitivity to allergens that the patient has been previously sensitized to.[27] This correlates with the pathogenesis of the disease, which is a type IV hypersensitivity immune response. By contrast, in ICD, the resulting inflammatory rash can occur within minutes to hours due to direct damage of keratinocytes by the irritant. It is related to the properties of the chemical itself rather than the immune-related process.[10,19] Here, the authors discuss the common types and causes of contact dermatitis that can be encountered in sports.

## CONTACT DERMATITIS

Contact dermatitis is often facilitated and exacerbated in sports by sweating into equipment, repetitive wetting, repeated drying, friction, and various chemicals that are used in different sport settings. An extensive review published by Kockentiet and Adams discusses in depth the different causes of contacts dermatitis in each sport.[19] Here, some of the more common conditions to be encountered by a primary care provider or sports trainer in the university or high school athletic setting are summarized.

### All Sports

- Topical benzocaine and lanolin, which are used in many topical medications and creams, have been reported to be one of the most common causes of ACD in sports.[7,10,19]

### Swimming

- Allergic
  - Goggles made with rubber or neoprene using benzoyl peroxide, phenol-formaldehyde resin, or various substituted thioureas have caused allergic dermatitis in areas of contact across the face.[17,28]
  - Mercaptobenzothiazole, which is found in some rubber bathing or swim caps, causes scalp dermatitis in swimmers.[19]
- Irritant and allergic
  - Disinfectant chemicals used in swimming pools, such as chlorinated compounds and bromides, have all been noted to cause both irritant and contact dermatitis.[19]

### Running

- Allergic
  - Topical therapeutic substances can induce ACD of the feet. It is important to ask if the patient is applying medications to the foot or spraying deodorizer into the shoes. Topical benzocaine and lanolin, which are used in many topical medications and creams, were reported to be the most common cause of ACD to the feet.[19]
- Irritant and allergic
  - It is common for athletes to react to rubber components in shoes, especially in the setting of sweat, as this causes increased skin exposure to the irritant. Because the insole has some of the highest contact with the foot, it is one of the most likely causes of dermatitis.[19,29]

### Soccer

- Allergic
  - Photolichenoid dermatitis has been reported due to plants that grow on the field. Shin guards have also been noted to cause ACD attributed to components of urea and formaldehyde.[19]
- Irritant and allergic
  - The lime component of the paint used for field markings has been implicated as a cause of ICD. This ICD characteristically occurs on the upper inner thighs, likely due to protection of the lower legs with socks and shin guards.[30,31]

### Tennis and Related Racket Sports

- Irritant and allergic
  - Rackets contain components such as isophorone diamine that can cause ACD. Neoprene splints used for tennis elbow have also been implicated. Rubber additives should always be considered in sports that use rubber balls and equipment, such as hand ball or squash.[19,29]

### Basketball

- Allergic
  - Rubber outdoor basketballs have caused ACD in some due to the rubber additives. ACD reactions to protective knee padding in basketball players have also been reported.[19,29]

*Hockey*

- Irritant and allergic
  - Fiberglass, a common component of hockey sticks, can lead to ICD. Epoxy resins in facemasks can result in facial ACD. Formaldehyde has also been reported as a causative agent due to its almost ubiquitous use in manufacturing sporting equipment, including hockey equipment.[19,29]

*Weightlifting*

- Irritant and allergic
  - Nickel is the most common positive finding on patch testing worldwide. It is sometimes used in weightlifting equipment and causes ACD. Chalk is another trigger of ICD that may affect some weightlifters who use it for grip.[19,29] Colophony (pine resin or resin) is allergenic and has been identified as causing dermatitis in weight lifters, as well as gymnasts and baseball pitchers.

*Evaluation and Management of Contact Dermatitis*

- Presentation
  - Patients often present with an erythematous, scaling, lichenified rash that is usually pruritic but may burn more if ICD is the main cause. They may also develop blistering if severe (**Fig. 10**). A rash can be generalized, such as in the setting of chlorine allergy, or localized, such as in rubber ingredients in goggles.[17,19,28]
- Diagnosis
  - History and physical examination can lead to the diagnoses of contact dermatitis. However, in order to determine the specific cause, patch testing may be necessary. It is helpful if a specific category of materials can be identified in the history to assist with testing.
- Prevention
  - After identifying the cause and determining irritant versus allergic, avoidance of the substances is the first-line treatment. Detailed information on product ingredients and safe products to use can be found at the American Contact Dermatitis Society Website www.contactderm.org and at www.dermatitisacademy.com.

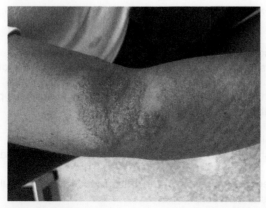

**Fig. 10.** Allergic contact dermatitis.

- Treatment
  - Medium to high potency topical steroids applied twice daily to affected areas can be helpful to control symptoms on the body. For thin areas of skin such as the axilla, groin, and face, mild potency steroids (hydrocortisone 2.5%) or calcineurin inhibitors (pimecrolimus, tacrolimus) are recommended. These areas have an increased risk of hypopigmentation and further skin thinning if medium to high strength topical steroids are used. If not controlled with topicals, referral to a dermatologist for initiation of systemic therapies is recommended.

## OTHER INFLAMMATORY DISORDERS
### Solar Urticaria

- Diagnosis and presentation[1,2]
  - Solar urticaria presents as itching and burning wheals with subsequent erythema, in sun-exposed areas that develop within minutes of exposure to sunlight or artificial ultraviolet B. Physical examination demonstrating urticaria in exposed skin with a history of it occurring shortly after sun exposure is sufficient for diagnosis. This condition tends to occur in the early summer and late spring months.
- Treatment
  - Antihistamines, sun protective clothing, sunscreen, and expectant management are usually sufficient. Hydroxychloroquine as well as Psoralen and ultraviolet A therapy can be helpful if symptoms are refractory.
- Prevention
  - Skin usually becomes less sensitive to the development of urticaria with repeated sun exposure. If this does not occur, covering sun-exposed areas is preventative. Sunscreen is generally not as effective as covering with clothing.

### Cholinergic Urticaria

- Diagnosis and presentation[2,10,28,32]
  - It presents as small wheals that develop shortly after exercise, usually after sweating begins. Development of urticaria after asking the patient to exercise is diagnostic.
- Treatment
  - Does not respond well to oral antihistamines, but it tends to resolve with age.
- Prevention
  - Avoiding exercise if antihistamines do not control symptoms.

### Cold Urticaria

- Diagnosis and presentation[2,23]
  - This occurs as small and large urticarial wheals in the areas of cold exposure, especially with cold-water contact. Presentation can also be generalized. Application of ice to the skin for 5 minutes is diagnostic if the patient develops wheals in the area.
- Treatment
  - Antihistamines can be helpful.
  - Patients should not swim alone due to risk of anaphylaxis resulting in drowning.
  - Rule out secondary causes of cold urticaria such as cryoglobulinemia and connective tissue disorders.
  - EpiPen should be provided.

- Prevention
  - Avoidance of cold weather.
  - Wearing protective clothing when exposed to cold environments.

## Infections in athletes

Skin infections are a common issue in sports dermatology due to close contact with other athletes, poor cleaning of equipment, environment, and trauma. Some of the infections that athletes are more prone to develop include bacterial soft tissue infections, tinea (dermatophyte fungal infection) of various types, hair follicle infections, and herpes. Some sport characteristics create opportunities for specific infections such as molluscum or herpes gladiatorum in wrestlers and pseudomonas folliculitis in swimmers. However, it has also been proposed that athletes are more prone to infections due to the suppressed immune barrier and trauma to the physical barrier by high intensity activites.[33] Overall, fungal infections tend to be the most common dermatologic infections experienced by athletes.[34] Because of the vast number of infections and their many possible associations to athletic events, this review of infections is not comprehensive; rather the authors present the most frequently encountered findings in the collegiate and high-school level of sports.

## BACTERIAL INFECTIONS
### Impetigo

- Diagnosis and presentation[4,35–38]
  - A very common and highly contagious superficial infection of the skin caused by staphylococcus or streptococcus species. Impetigo can be spread through skin-to-skin contact either through small breaks in the skin or in untraumatized skin. It usually presents with papules and vesicles coalescing into a plaque with an overlying honey-colored crust (**Fig. 11**). History and physical examination can often lead to the diagnosis; however, cultures of the lesion can aid in the diagnosis.
- Treatment
  - Removal of the overlying crust and treatment with topical mupirocin is often sufficient for mild infections. First-generation cephalosporins or macrolides are effective for more severe infections. If culture reveals methicillin-resistant *Staphylococcus aureus* (MRSA), appropriate change of coverage in antibiotics may be needed.
- Prevention
  - Avoiding skin contact with infected individuals as well as avoiding sharing of unwashed equipment, clothes, or towels are important. Furthermore, any open wounds should be kept clean with dry bandages and twice-daily application of triple antibiotics or mupirocin should be done until the wound is no longer open.

### Bacterial Folliculitis

- Diagnosis and presentation[2,35,37,39]
  - This presents as inflammation within the superficial portion of the hair follicle that can be caused by multiple infectious causes. It usually occurs as inflamed pustular papules in a follicular distribution (**Fig. 12**). Infectious agents include staphylococcus and pseudomonas, with staphylococcus being the most common cause of folliculitis. It can present in any area of the body but is often found in occluded areas, is frequently painful, and mildly pruritic. Alternatively,

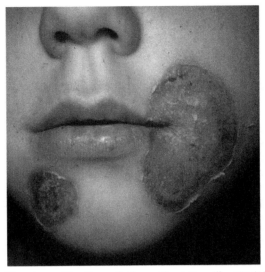

**Fig. 11.** Impetigo. (*Courtesy of* Dr. Kenneth Greer Charlottesville, Virginia.)

pseudomonas folliculitis occurs from poorly cleaned bathtubs, hot tubs, and whirlpools. It, too, usually crops up in occluded areas such as under bathing suits or in axillary folds. History can be helpful in diagnosis. If there exists a recent hot tub or possible contaminated water source exposure, consider pseudomonas, otherwise staphylococcus folliculitis should be highest on the differential. Cultures of pustules can be helpful for differentiation but are often not necessary.

- Treatment
  - For methicillin-susceptible *S aureus* (MSSA), oral antibiotics such as cephalosporins or macrolides are effective. For MRSA, treatment with doxycycline or sulfamethoxazole/trimethoprim is recommended.
  - For Pseudomonas, treatment with oral antibiotics is often not helpful, becuase the folliculitis is self-limiting over 5 to 7 days. However, for severe or recalcitrant infections, some recommend treatment with oral fluoroquinolones.

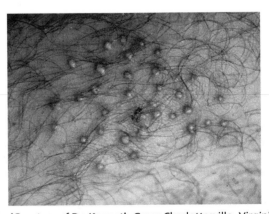

**Fig. 12.** Folliculitis. (*Courtesy of* Dr. Kenneth Greer Charlottesville, Virginia.)

- Prevention
  - Keeping equipment clean and avoiding the sharing of towels with other athletes is a helpful prevention tactic. Others include bathing with antibacterial soap immediately after sport activities and only using regularly cleaned hot tubs.

## Abscesses and Furuncles

- Diagnosis and presentation[2,10,35–38]
  - Abscesses and furuncles usually present as erythematous, painful, and fluctuant nodules. They commonly occur in occluded areas in the folds of the skin yet can appear in areas of repeated trauma between equipment and skin, which results in friction. For mild infections, there are no systemic symptoms such as fever and chills. History and physical examination is classically sufficient for diagnosis. Blood cultures are helpful for antibiotic guidance; however, the vast majority is caused by staphylococcus species. The main goal of cultures, if indicated, is to rule out MRSA. Collecting the history of risk factors proves helpful as well.
- Treatment
  - For small, mild cases that do not cause severe symptoms, warm compresses and antibiotics can be sufficient. However, larger lesions or very symptomatic lesions will require incision and drainage for treatment. If the abscess is very large, a drain may be required to prevent incision closure and thus reoccurrence of the abscess.
- Prevention
  - Cleaning open wounds with antibacterial soap and keeping them covered with topical antibiotics can prevent occurrence of deeper infections.

## Cellulitis and Erysipelas

- Diagnosis and presentation[7,10,36–38,40]
  - Patients will often present with a well-defined area of erythema, edema, and pain that characterizes these diseases. Erysipelas is characterized by infection of the superficial layers of the skin classically on the face (**Fig. 13**). Cellulitis is defined as infection that involves the subcutaneous layers of the skin. These symptoms can be accompanied by fever; however, the absence of fever does not rule out the diagnosis. These infections are most commonly caused by group A streptococcus and staphylococcus species. History of quickly spreading unilateral erythema, fevers, and pain, along with a physical examination demonstrating unilateral pain to palpation with associated skin warmth is adequate for the diagnosis. Blood cultures are helpful for systemic or severe symptoms.
- Treatment
  - Antibiotics are a mainstay of treatment with choice of MRSA coverage based on the local prevalence and patient risk factors. MRSA systemic coverage include sulfamethoxazole/trimethoprim and doxycycline. Options of MSSA or streptococcus include cephalosporins and macrolides. Severe symptoms or cellulitis that involves large areas warrant intravenous antibiotics and hospital admission.
- Prevention
  - Minimizing skin trauma or skin damage as well as good wound care help with prevention.

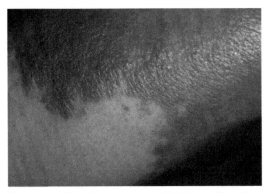

**Fig. 13.** Erysipelas. (*Courtesy of* Dr. Kenneth Greer Charlottesville, Virginia.)

### Pitted Keratolysis

- Diagnosis and presentation[2,23,35]
  - Pitted keratolysis presents with hyperhidrosis, striking malodor, and skin sliminess with characteristic pitting of the soles of the feet (**Fig. 14**). This is commonly found on the pressure-bearing areas of the feet. Pathogenesis is related to a proliferation of bacteria such as corynebacterium species that secrete keratinase. History and physical examination demonstrating the characteristic findings stated earlier will lead to diagnosis.
- Treatment
  - Every effort should be made to keep the area dry by changing out socks regularly. Eliminating moisture generally treats the infection. Using antiperspirant medication in the area can also prove helpful. Antibiotic therapy with topical 2% erythromycin or 1% clindamycin will treat refractory cases.
- Prevention
  - Keeping feet dry and avoiding prolonged moisture is effective in prevention. Selecting synthetic rather than cotton socks and using aluminum chloride-based antiperspirants are other preventive actions.

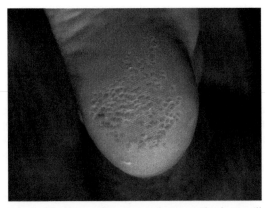

**Fig. 14.** Pitted keratolysis. (*Courtesy of* Dr. Kenneth Greer Charlottesville, Virginia.)

### Erythrasma

- Diagnosis and presentation[10,35,41]
  - ○ Erythrasma normally presents in warm, moist areas of the foot with erythematous, thin, wet plaques (**Fig. 15**). This develops due to the effects of corynebacterium in warm and humid environments of skin creases such as between toes, in the axilla, and in the groin. Physical examination will indicate the disease; however, coral red fluorescence under wood lamp can help with the diagnosis. If Gram stain is performed, it will show gram-positive, rod-shaped organisms.
- Treatment
  - ○ Topical erythromycin or clindamycin applied twice daily for 14 days is generally effective. Oral regimens include doxycycline, erythromycin, or clarithromycin.
- Prevention
  - ○ Good hygiene and keeping creases and folds of the skin dry when possible help to prevent reinfection.

## VIRAL INFECTIONS
### Molluscum

- Diagnosis and presentation[37]
  - ○ Molluscum presents as skin-colored, dome-shaped papules that can be umbilicated in the center. Any area of skin that comes into contact with another infected athlete can be affected, and this is a particular problem for wrestlers. Diagnosis may be made on history and physical examination alone.
- Treatment
  - ○ Treatment is focused on irritation of the lesion to induce a response by the patient's immune system. Cryotherapy and curettage are used most often. Topical retinoids are another option.
- Prevention
  - ○ Avoiding contact with infected individuals and wearing appropriate protective clothes and equipment in areas that may be exposed are good practices for prevention.

### Herpes Simplex

- Diagnosis and presentation[1,14,37,42]
  - ○ Herpes simplex manifests as grouped vesicles with an erythematous base (**Fig. 16**). Although often associated as a sexually transmitted disease in genital

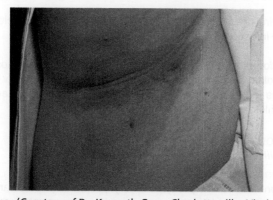

**Fig. 15.** Erythrasma. (*Courtesy of* Dr. Kenneth Greer Charlottesville, Virginia.)

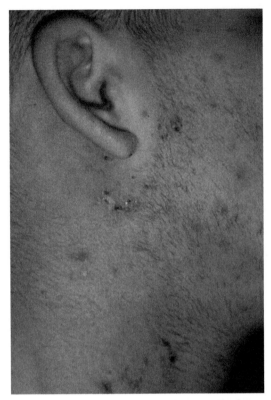

**Fig. 16.** Herpes gladiatorum. (*Courtesy of* Dr. Kenneth Greer Charlottesville, Virginia.)

areas, it can occur in any area of skin that comes into contact with an actively infected, moist rash of another player. Herpes gladiatorum is a specific eruption in wrestlers and results from the skin (often cheek or neck) of a wrestler coming into contact with another wrestler's infected skin during common wrestling maneuvers. Physical examination of grouped vesicles on an erythematous base can lead to diagnosis and a Tzanck smear providing confirmation if needed. For more specific and sensitive tests, polymerase chain reaction, viral cultures, or direct immunofluorescence antibodies are available.

- Treatment
  - Oral antiviral agents such as acyclovir, valacyclovir, or famciclovir are effective for active infection.
- Prevention
  - Examination of wrestlers, or "skin checks," before competition is required by most scholastic and collegiate wrestling federations to identify herpetic lesions (as well as molluscum and tinea). Avoiding skin-to-skin contact with other infected athletes prevents infection.

## FUNGAL INFECTIONS
### Pityrosporum Folliculitis

- Diagnosis and presentation[17]
  - Pityrosporum folliculitis presents as erythematous papules and pustules in a follicular pattern that tends to occur on the upper trunk and proximal upper

extremities (**Fig. 17**). It is often misdiagnosed as bacterial folliculitis or acne. This classically occurs during the summer months in the setting of significant heat, sweating, and poor personal hygiene habits.

- Treatment
  - ○ Ketoconazole and selenium sulfide shampoo applied twice weekly are effective topical treatments. Oral treatment options include itraconazole or ketoconazole; however, side effects of oral medications should be considered.
- Prevention
  - ○ Prophylactic topical ketoconazole shampoo can be effective for some patients.

### Tinea

- Diagnosis and presentation[10,14,18,43,44]
  - ○ Tinea normally presents as an erythematous, mildly scaly annular papule or plaque with a raised edge and central clearing (**Fig. 18**). It can infect most areas of the body, especially areas that come into contact with the skin of other infected athletes.
- Diagnosis
  - ○ Physical examination and microscopic potassium hydroxide skin preparation examination of scrapings from the lesion will demonstrate hyphae and other fungal elements.
- Treatment
  - ○ Topical or oral antifungal medication such as oral terbinafine, oral or topical fluconazole, or topical ketoconazole.

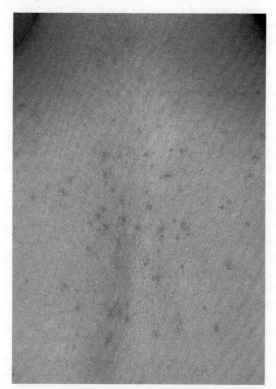

**Fig. 17.** Pityrosporum folliculitis. (*Courtesy of* Dr. Kenneth Greer Charlottesville, Virginia.)

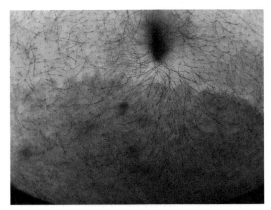

**Fig. 18.** Tinea corporis. (*Courtesy of* Dr. Darren Guffey Charlottesville, Virginia.)

- Prevention
  - In severe outbreaks among teams, prophylactic antifungals can be beneficial; however, intense surveillance of athletes can also help in prevention.

## SUMMARY

Athletic skin disorders typically fall into 3 categories: mechanical skin injury, inflammatory skin conditions, and infectious skin conditions. The athletic trainer is frequently confronted with a wide variety of these skin conditions. The trainer's knowledge of equipment and conditions encountered by the athlete provides important insight into potential causes and treatment of these conditions.

## REFERENCES

1. Helm TN, Bergfeld WF. Sports dermatology. Clin Dermatol 1998;16(1):159–65.
2. Pharis DB, Teller C, Wolf JE. Cutaneous manifestations of sports participation. J Am Acad Dermatol 1997;36(3):448–59.
3. Herring K, Richie D. Friction blisters and sock fiber composition. A double-blind study. J Am Podiatr Med Assoc 1990;80(2):63–71.
4. Adams BB. Dermatologic disorders of the athlete. Sports Med 2002;32(5): 309–21.
5. Heymann WR. Dermatologic problems of the endurance athlete. J Am Acad Dermatol 2005;52(2):345–6.
6. Mailler EA, Adams BB. The wear and tear of 26.2: dermatological injuries reported on marathon day. Br J Sports Med 2004;38(4):498–501.
7. Farhadian JA, Tlougan BE, Adams BB, et al. Skin conditions of baseball, cricket, and softball players. Sports Med 2013;43(7):575–89.
8. Vogt T, Brunnberg S, Hohenleutner U, et al. Bullous malignant melanoma: an unusual differential diagnosis of a hemorrhagic friction blister. Dermatol Surg 2003; 29(1):102–4.
9. Zarâa I, Trojjet S, Mokni M, et al. Dermatologic disorders of the athlete: a report of 30 cases? Tunis Med 2008;86(10):865–8 [in French].
10. Emer J, Sivek R, Marciniak B. Sports dermatology: part 1 of 2 traumatic or mechanical injuries, inflammatory conditions, and exacerbations of pre-existing conditions. J Clin Aesthet Dermatol 2015;8(4):31–43.

11. Cordoro KM, Ganz JE. Training room management of medical conditions: sports dermatology. Clin Sports Med 2005;24(3):565–98.

12. Basler RSW. Skin injuries in sports medicine. J Am Acad Dermatol 1989;21(6): 1257–62.

13. Bae JM, Kang H, Kim HO, et al. Differential diagnosis of plantar wart from corn, callus and healed wart with the aid of dermoscopy. Br J Dermatol 2009;160(1): 220–2.

14. De Luca JF, Adams BB, Yosipovitch G. Skin manifestations of athletes competing in the summer olympics. Sports Med 2012;42(5):399–413.

15. Mailler-Savage EA, Adams BB. Skin manifestations of running. J Am Acad Dermatol 2006;55(2):290–301.

16. Descamps V, Claessens Y-E, Doumenc B. Skin manifestations in ultramarathon runners: experience in the Marathon des Sables 2014. Br J Dermatol 2017; 177(2):562–3.

17. Freiman A, Barankin B, Elpern DJ. Sports dermatology part 1: common dermatoses. CMAJ 2004;171(8):851–3.

18. Metelitsa A, Barankin B, Lin AN. Diagnosis of sports-related dermatoses. Int J Dermatol 2004;43(2):113–9.

19. Kockentiet B, Adams BB. Contact dermatitis in athletes. J Am Acad Dermatol 2007;56(6):1048–55.

20. Ashman CJ, Klecker RJ, Yu JS. Forefoot pain involving the metatarsal region: differential diagnosis with MR imaging. Radiographics 2001;21(6):1425–40.

21. Cohen PR, Eliezri YD, Silvers DN. Athlete's nodules. J Am Acad Dermatol 1991; 24(2):317–8.

22. Conklin RJ. Common cutaneous disorders in athletes. Sports Med 1990;9(2): 100–19.

23. Tlougan BE, Podjasek JO, Adams BB. Aquatic sports dermatoses: part 1. in the water: freshwater dermatoses. Int J Dermatol 2010;49(8):874–85.

24. Chan C-C, Chiu H-C. Erythema Ab Igne. N Engl J Med 2007;356(9):e8.

25. Sigmon JR, Cantrell J, Teague D, et al. Poorly differentiated carcinoma arising in the setting of erythema Ab Igne. Am J Dermatopathol 2013;35(6):676–8.

26. Clark SC, Zirwas MJ. Management of occupational dermatitis. Dermatol Clin 2009;27(3):365–83, vii-viii.

27. Beltrani VS. The clinical spectrum of atopic dermatitis. J Allergy Clin Immunol 1999;104(3 Pt 2):S87–98.

28. Del Giacco SR, Manconi PE, Del Giacco GS. Allergy and sports. Allergy 2001; 56(3):215–23.

29. Brooks CD, Kujawska A, Patel D. Cutaneous allergic reactions induced by sporting activities. Sports Med 2003;33(9):699–708.

30. Fisher AA. Cement injuries. Part III: Cement burns in soccer and rugby players. Cutis 1998;61(4):182.

31. Mastrolonardo M, Cassano N, Veña GA. Cement burns in 2 football players. Contact Dermatitis 1997;37(4):183–4.

32. Macucci F, Guerrini L, Strambi M. Asthma and allergy in young athletes in Siena Province. Preliminary results. J Sports Med Phys Fitness 2007;47(3):351–5.

33. Eda N, Shimizu K, Suzuki S, et al. Effects of high-intensity endurance exercise on epidermal barriers against microbial invasion. J Sports Sci Med 2013;12(1): 44–51.

34. Derya A, Ilgen E, Metin E. Characteristics of sports-related dermatoses for different types of sports: a cross-sectional study. J Dermatol 2005;32(8):620–5.

35. Adams BB. Skin infections in athletes. In: Hall BJ, Hall JC, editors. Skin infections: diagnosis and treatment. Cambridge Medicine; 2009. p. 238–46.

36. Cohen PR. The skin in the gym: a comprehensive review of the cutaneous manifestations of community-acquired methicillin-resistant Staphylococcus aureus infection in athletes. Clin Dermatol 2008;26(1):16–26.

37. Likness LP. Common dermatologic infections in athletes and return-to-play guidelines. J Am Osteopath Assoc 2011;111(6):373.

38. Kirkland EB, Adams BB. Methicillin-resistant Staphylococcus aureus and athletes. J Am Acad Dermatol 2008;59(3):494–502.

39. Adams BB. Skin infections in athletes. Dermatol Nurs 2008;20(1):39–44.

40. Tlougan BE, Podjasek JO, Adams BB. Review: aquatic sports dematoses. Part 2 - in the water: saltwater dermatoses. Int J Dermatol 2010;49(9):994–1002.

41. Pecci M, Comeau D, Chawla V. Skin conditions in the athlete. Am J Sports Med 2009;37(2):406–18.

42. Belongia EA, Goodman JL, Holland EJ, et al. An outbreak of herpes gladiatorum at a high-school wrestling camp. N Engl J Med 1991;325(13):906–10.

43. Purim KSM, Bordignon GPF, Queiroz-Telles F de. Fungal infection of the feet in soccer players and non-athlete individuals. Rev Iberoam Micol 2005;22(1):34–8.

44. Pleacher MD, Dexter WW. Cutaneous fungal and viral infections in athletes. Clin Sports Med 2007;26(3):397–411.

# Training Room Procedures and Use of Therapeutic Modalities in Athletes

Siobhan Statuta, MD[a,b,*], Kelli Pugh, MS, ATC, LMT[c]

## KEYWORDS

- Therapeutic modalities • Manual therapy • Musculoskeletal injury • Laceration • Nail
- Auricular

## KEY POINTS

- Athletic trainers and physical therapists use various therapeutic modalities and manual therapies as an adjunct to rehabilitation exercises to enhance recovery from injury.
- Clinicians should be knowledgeable of the current literature to determine the most efficacious use of therapeutic modalities, based on the type of injury and stage of healing.
- When managing acute injuries in the training room, physicians must understand what the crucial components of the history and physical examination findings are to guide the appropriate intervention.

Athletic trainers and physical therapists use a variety of therapeutic modalities in the treatment of surgical and nonsurgical musculoskeletal injuries. These modalities are used to relieve pain, decrease swelling and/or stiffness, and modify the body's inflammatory response to promote healing so that the patient may more effectively perform rehabilitation exercises. Commonly used modalities include cryotherapy, thermotherapy, therapeutic ultrasound, electrical stimulation, compression devices, and soft tissue manipulation. The sports medicine clinician should be confident in choosing the appropriate modality based on the patient's level of inflammation and stage of recovery.

The authors have no disclosures or conflict of interest.
[a] Primary Care Sports Medicine Fellowship, Department of Family Medicine, University of Virginia Sports Medicine, University of Virginia Health System, Charlottesville, VA, USA; [b] Primary Care Sports Medicine Fellowship, Department of Physical Medicine and Rehabilitation, University of Virginia Sports Medicine, University of Virginia Health System, Charlottesville, VA, USA; [c] University of Virginia, 290 Massie Road, Room 112, Charlottesville, VA 22904, USA
* Corresponding author. Primary Care Sports Medicine Fellowship, Department of Family Medicine, University of Virginia Sports Medicine, University of Virginia Health System, Charlottesville, VA.
E-mail address: siobhan@virginia.edu

## CRYOTHERAPY

Ice is frequently recommended as an initial treatment after an acute musculoskeletal injury and as a means of encouraging recovery from sports activity. The physiologic effects of cold include decreases in pain, blood flow, inflammation, edema, tissue metabolic demand, and muscle spasm.[1,2] Dupuy and colleagues[3] reported that only immersion in water temperatures below 15°C (59°F) had a positive impact on muscle damage and inflammation as measured by changes in creatine kinase, IL-6, and C-reactive protein. Cold water immersion has been shown to significantly decrease the subjective symptoms of delayed onset muscle soreness.[4]

Although readily available and commonly used, this modality still requires informed clinical judgment before application.[5]

- *Indications:* decrease pain, decrease muscle spasm, limit swelling through vasoconstriction, decrease injury to secondary tissues by decreasing metabolic demand, recovery from exertion
- *Contraindications:* Raynaud's phenomenon, cold urticaria
- *Precautions:* decreased sensation, direct application over superficial nerves, poor local circulation, slow-healing wounds

Cryotherapy can take several forms, with advantages and disadvantages to each type (**Figs. 1** and **2, Table 1**).

## THERMOTHERAPY

Thermotherapy refers to any therapeutic modality designed to increase tissue temperature. Superficial heating modalities produce changes in skin temperature, but have little impact on deeper tissues.[5] Despite these limited effects, heat is frequently preferred by patients and commonly used in athletic training and physical therapy settings. When applied safely and appropriately, superficial heat can be a helpful modality before therapeutic exercise.[2,5]

- *Indications:* decrease pain, decrease muscle spasm
- *Contraindications:* acute injury, diminished sensation, poor local circulation, active swelling
- *Precautions:* medically unstable, coronary heart disease

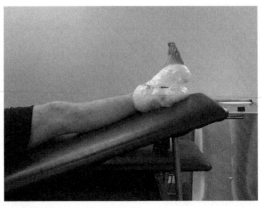

**Fig. 1.** An ice bag is applied to a patient's ankle.

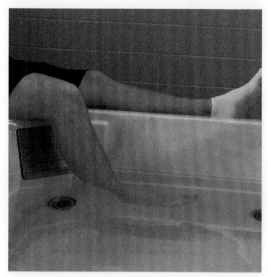

**Fig. 2.** A patient performs ankle range of motion exercises while in cold water immersion.

Superficial thermotherapy can take many forms, with advantages and disadvantages to each type (**Fig. 3, Table 2**). Therapeutic ultrasound is a deep heating modality is discussed further in the ultrasound section of this article.

## CONTRAST WATER THERAPY

Contrast baths involve alternating extremity or full body immersion in hot and cold water. It provides a strong sensory effect to the patient, meaning the hot feels hotter

| Table 1 | | |
| --- | --- | --- |
| **Therapeutic modalities: advantages and disadvantages of forms of cryotherapy** | | |
| **Form of Cryotherapy** | **Advantages** | **Disadvantages** |
| Ice bag | Moldable to the injured area Allows for simultaneous elevation Can wrap treatment "to go" after activity Cost efficient | Must use care postoperatively or with open wounds, because the melting ice could get wounds wet Sometimes difficult to perform simultaneous range of motion exercises |
| Cold water immersion | Allows for simultaneous range of motion exercise | Contraindicated postoperatively or with open wounds Gravity-dependent position not advised for patients with considerable swelling |
| Commercial cold water circulating unit | Keeps postoperative wounds dry Allows for simultaneous elevation and compression | More expensive Must have individual wraps per body part Difficult to perform simultaneous range of motion exercise owing to restriction from the wrap |

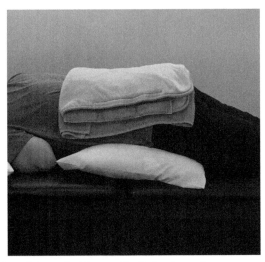

**Fig. 3.** A moist hot pack is applied to a patient's lumbar spine.

and the cold feels colder. Full body contrast water therapy is frequently used as a means of recovery from strenuous exercise. Bieuzen and colleagues[6] confirmed that contrast therapy induces successive peripheral vasoconstriction and vasodilation, but found no difference in terms of subjective muscle soreness compared with cold water immersion. However, contrast therapy did significantly decrease muscle soreness compared with warm water immersion recovery. Dupuy and colleagues[3] reported decreased creatine kinase concentrations in the blood after contrast water therapy, indicating decreased muscle damage. The same indications and contraindications for cold and warm water immersion apply respectively for contrast water therapy application.

**Table 2**
**Therapeutic modalities: advantages and disadvantages of forms of thermotherapy**

| Form of Superficial Thermotherapy | Advantages | Disadvantages |
|---|---|---|
| Moist heat pack | Easy application<br>Patient convenience (keeps patient dry) | Limited size of treatment area |
| Warm water immersion | Allows for heating of large areas<br>Movement of the water massages the tissue<br>Allows for simultaneous range of motion exercise | Contraindicated postoperatively or with open wounds |
| Paraffin bath | Allows for heating of the entire area submerged, good for distal extremities | Contraindicated postoperatively or with open wounds<br>Application limited to distal extremities, based on size of the bath<br>Cannot perform simultaneous range of motion exercise |

## THERAPEUTIC ULTRASOUND

Therapeutic ultrasound is used frequently by athletic trainers and physical therapists in the treatment of musculoskeletal injuries such as sprains, strains, tendinopathy, and bursitis. This modality uses acoustic energy, delivered at very specific high frequencies, to create thermal or nonthermal changes in tissue. An electrical current, configured by the parameters set by the clinician, creates a mechanical vibration in the crystalline material in the attached sound head. The vibration of the crystal produces sounds waves that are transmitted through a coupling medium to the target tissue.[5] Frequency parameters can be adjusted to treat superficial or deeper structures.

Thermal ultrasound can be used as a deep heating modality, with the ability to reach ligament, joint capsule, muscle, tendon, and scar tissue. The therapeutic benefits of continuous ultrasound are similar to other heating modalities, including decreased muscle spasm and joint stiffness while also causing increased collagen extensibility and blood flow.[2] In addition to warming the target tissue, the treatment area receives the nonthermal effects of ultrasound. The clinician can adjust the duty cycle parameter of the treatment to a pulsed setting, thereby interrupting the delivery of the sound wave. This feature makes ultrasound therapy appropriate for use with acute injuries by eliminating the thermal effects. The nonthermal effects of ultrasound facilitate repair of the injured tissue through the increased movement of fluid and dissolved nutrients to and across cell membranes. This movement is caused by acoustic streaming and stable cavitation[5] (**Box 1**). Therapeutic benefits of pulsed ultrasound include reduction of inflammatory infiltrates and exudates and decreased edema[2] (**Fig. 4**).

- *Indications*
  - ○ Continuous duty cycle (thermal effects): subacute or chronic injury, with the goal of heating deeper tissue and increasing blood flow
  - ○ Pulsed duty cycle (nonthermal effects): acute injury, with the goal of facilitating the healing environment in the tissues
- *Contraindications:* cancer; infection; application over cardiac pacemaker, eyes, genitalia, and joint replacements; minimize exposure over open epiphyses and spinal cord

Despite its widespread use, the literature is mixed on the efficacy of therapeutic ultrasound. Lengthy treatment durations are required to achieve substantial change in tissue temperature. Desmeules and colleagues[7] reported no benefit of ultrasound compared with placebo and no added benefit when combined with exercise for treatment of rotator cuff tendinopathy. Shanks and colleagues[8] also found no high-quality evidence to support the use of ultrasound for musculoskeletal conditions of the lower extremity. However, there is strong evidence in animal studies supporting the effects of therapeutic ultrasound on tendon healing.[9] Ultrasound can have a positive effect on collagen synthesis by stimulating cell migration and proliferation, which may benefit

---

**Box 1**
**Therapeutic modalities**

Nonthermal effects of therapeutic ultrasound
- Acoustical streaming: The movement of fluids along cell membranes owing to the mechanical pressure of the sound waves.
- Stable cavitation: Gas bubbles are formed due to pressure changes in the tissue. The rhythmic expansion and contraction of these bubbles facilitates fluid movement and membrane transport.

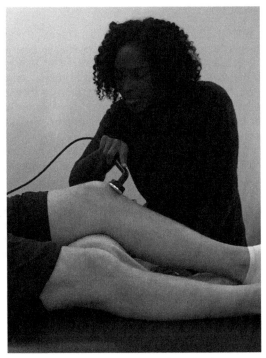

**Fig. 4.** An athletic trainer performs therapeutic ultrasound on a patient with patellar tendinitis.

tendon healing. Clinicians must follow the recommended treatment parameters of frequency, duty cycle, and intensity to gain therapeutic benefit from a treatment that may otherwise be placebo.

## PHONOPHORESIS

Phonophoresis describes using sound energy to drive medication (commonly some form of antiinflammatory medication) through the patient's skin. Clinicians must ensure the active ingredient is mixed in a gel that is a known conductor of acoustic energy. It is difficult to determine when a pharmacologically effective dose has been administered. The efficacy of phonophoresis varies depending on the condition being treated and the medication administered.

## BONE STIMULATORS

Physicians occasionally prescribe low-intensity pulsed ultrasound stimulators (LIPUS) to patients with a fracture in an attempt to speed the bone healing process. These simulators are costly and frequently not covered by health insurance. In animal and in vitro studies, LIPUS seems to improve the bone healing response. In humans, LIPUS seems to be more effective in the treatment of delayed nonunion fractures or in patients with comorbidities that could affect fracture healing, such as advanced age, malnourishment, diabetes, or smoking.[10] Schandelmaier and colleagues[11] reported moderate evidence that LIPUS have no effect on radiographic healing in patients with acute fracture or osteotomy. In addition to LIPUS bone stimulators, there are also pulsed electromagnetic field bone stimulators. These devices have demonstrated usefulness in the healing of nonunion fractures.[5] Clinicians should consider the type of fracture and the cost–benefit implications for each patient before prescribing such devices as a part of fracture management.

## ELECTRICAL STIMULATION

Transcutaneous electrical nerve stimulation (TENS) is another commonly encountered therapeutic modality that applies an electrical current to target specific tissues in the body. Depending on the parameters of the type of current applied and dosage, TENS can be used to achieve a variety of clinical goals[2,5] (**Fig. 5**).

- *Indications:* pain relief, muscle stimulation, stimulation of denervated muscle, iontophoresis, edema reduction, and wound healing
- *Contraindications:* electrode placement over carotid artery, cardiac pacemaker, pregnancy

Portable TENS units have become affordable and available to the general public and offer a convenient, nonpharmacologic form of pain management. In the athletic training or physical therapy setting, TENS is also commonly used in conjunction with ice or heat to combine treatment goals of pain relief or edema reduction with the desired effect of the other respective modality.

### *Iontophoresis*

Iontophoresis uses a direct electrical current to deliver medication to a target tissue. It is based on the principal that like electrical charges are repelled and provides a noninvasive method of local drug administration.[2,5] Dexamethasone is regularly used in athletic training settings to suppress inflammation in superficial tissues. Although widely available, iontophoresis seems to be most effective for short-term, rapid reduction in pain after an acute injury.[2] Because iontophoresis involves the use of prescription medication, athletic trainers and physical therapists should consult their state practice act to determine what physician oversight is required to administer iontophoresis.

- *Indications:* acute inflammation in superficial tissues
- *Contraindications:* same as TENS—allergy or sensitivity to the prescribed medication

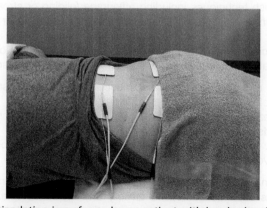

**Fig. 5.** Electrical stimulation is performed on a patient with low back pain.

## COMPRESSION

The application of compression to limit local swelling and edema after an acute injury is a well-established treatment method. Compression has been popularized as a means of recovery from strenuous exercise and is a common modality found in the athletic training and physical therapy setting.

### Pneumatic Compression Device

Commercial units use compressed air to provide compression through an extremity-specific wrap or sleeve. These units can provide either focal or sequential compression, depending on the design of the attachment. Pneumatic compression devices have been used in postoperative and stroke patients as a means of deep vein thrombosis prophylaxis. Haun and colleagues[12] found that pneumatic compression devices used after repeated bouts of high-intensity interval training decreased evidence of skeletal muscle markers of proteolysis. Winke and Williamson[13] reported pneumatic compression device use provided decreased muscle swelling, decreased peak pain, and less disturbance in range of motion compared with the use of compression garments in the treatment of delayed onset muscle soreness.

### Compression Garments

Compression garments have been marketed by athletic clothing companies as a means of promoting recovery after exercise. These garments vary in their size (extremity vs whole body) and the amount of pressure applied. There are no set treatment parameters for duration of use. Although there are conflicting results on objective measures of muscle damage and inflammation after the use of compression garmets,[3,14] it has been shown that their use can have a significant and positive impact on decreasing fatigue and the perception of delayed onset muscle soreness.[3] Brown and colleagues[15] reported compression garments were most effective for enhancing recovery after resistance exercise.

## MANUAL THERAPY TECHNIQUES
### Massage

Massage has been used for thousands of years to promote soft tissue recovery and healing. Athletic trainers and physical therapists use massage as a part of the treatment plan for musculoskeletal injuries, to prepare a patient or athlete for exercise, to enhance athletic performance, and to promote recovery from strenuous exercise.[16] Traditional Swedish techniques including effleurage (gliding or stroking), petrissage (kneading), friction, and tapotement (tapping) are the basis of most massage therapies. Varieties of myofascial techniques have been developed to address specific musculoskeletal complaints. These techniques use a combination of slower strokes and static holds at moderate depth to influence trigger points or fascia.

- *Indications:* reducing pain, edema, muscle tension or spasm, anxiety, and perception of fatigue; promoting relaxation
- *Contraindications:* fever, acute illness, malignancies, regional skin conditions or open wounds
- *Precautions:* arteriosclerosis, hematomas, hypotension, osteoporosis, phlebitis, postoperatively

The effects of massage are most likely achieved by more than one mechanism. Psychological effects such as decreased anxiety and increased relaxation are likely derived through activation of the parasympathetic nervous system. Biomechanical and physiologic effects are achieved through mechanical manipulation of the tissue, causing increased muscle blood flow and peripheral circulation, decreased tissue adhesion, decreased passive and active stiffness, and increased joint range of motion. Neurologic effects are caused by reflex stimulation, resulting in decreased pain, muscle tension and spasm, and neuromuscular excitability.[17,18]

### Instrumented Soft Tissue Manipulation

Instrumented soft tissue manipulation uses specially designed instruments to mobilize the soft tissue in the treatment of injuries or myofascial restrictions. These instruments vary in material and shape based on the company producing them. Instrumented soft tissue manipulation provides athletic trainers and physical therapists with a method of manual therapy that decreases strain on the clinician (**Fig. 6**). Because of inconsistent instrument choice and methodology in emerging instrumented soft tissue manipulation research, there is no consensus on whether this method is more or less effective than manual massage.

### Cupping

Whereas massage applies mechanical pressure to the tissues, myofascial decompression, commonly known as cupping therapy, applies suction to the skin through the use of a hollow container. Cupping is another ancient modality that has been used around the world for thousands of years. Wet cupping involves the use of a needle or scalpel to pierce the skin before the application of the cup and suction. In

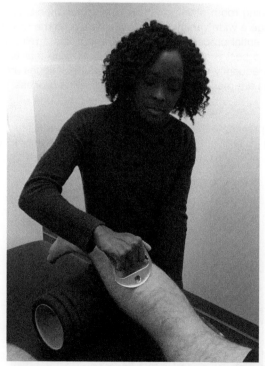

**Fig. 6.** An athletic trainer performs instrumented soft tissue manipulation on a patient's hamstring.

current Western medical practice, dry cupping is performed with plastic cups and a hand or electric pump to create suction to the skin. Soft silicone cups can also be applied where the suction is created by hand[19,20] (**Fig. 7**). It is expected for dry cupping to leave a circular, sometimes ecchymotic, cupping mark. Moving or dynamic cupping involves sliding a cup along the skin after placement with light suction.

The effects of cupping are varied and not well-explained by a single rationale. Cupping has been used with varying levels of evidence in the treatment of migraines, musculoskeletal pain, carpal tunnel syndrome, and fibromyalgia, in addition to many other primary care conditions such as asthma, acne, cough, and urticaria.[19,20] For musculoskeletal conditions, cupping increases blood flow to the skin and muscles, decreases pain, and stimulates the peripheral nervous system.[20] Although cupping sets are readily available for relatively low prices, clinicians should receive training in this modality before application on patients.

### Dry Needling

Dry needling describes the insertion of thin monofilament needles, such as those used in acupuncture, in the treatment of myofascial trigger points. It is indicated for short-term decreases of pain and decreased muscle spasm in myofascial pain conditions. Needles can be placed alone, applied in conjunction with electrical stimulation, or used in a repeated in-and-out technique called pistoning or pecking.[21] Athletic trainers and physical therapists should consult their state practice act on training requirements and permissions required before performing dry needling.

### TRAINING ROOM PROCEDURES

In the athletic training room physician clinic, the sports medicine provider must be prepared to manage a wide variety of acute conditions, some of which may present the need for a potential procedure. Although there exists a relative paucity of new evidence relating to best practices, it is nevertheless wise that each physician feel comfortable with frequently encountered procedural techniques and ensure that the necessary supplies are readily available to streamline the process.

### Laceration Repair

Athletes regularly present to the athletic training room urgently after having sustained a laceration from a collision or fall. Indications for closure include hemostasis,

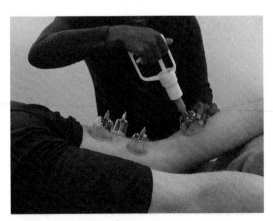

**Fig. 7.** Cupping is applied on a patient's leg.

decreasing the risk of infection, and providing the patient with the best possible cosmetic result.[22] Ideally, this is managed expeditiously because wound closure within less than 12 to 18 hours yields the most favorable results.[22,23] As such, it is helpful for any health care provider working in the setting of an athletic training room to be comfortable with acceptable methods of closure as well as possible complications.

## Evaluation

Before any repair, it is important to obtain a thorough history of how the injury occurred and a detailed assessment of the wound. Critical components of the history include mechanism of injury, the setting in which it occurred, time elapsed since the injury, and other indicators that raise suspicion for other, less obvious but concerning conditions such as internal bleeding or concussion. Tetanus status, current medications, and a review of allergies should also be obtained. The wound must then be explored carefully, taking note of the shape, size, depth, and location.[22,23]

Not all lacerations should be repaired in the athletic training room with complicated cases referred for further assessment and possible surgical consult. These include lacerations involving vessels, bone, tendons, joints, nerves or for any full-thickness laceration of the lip, ear, or eyelid.[22,23] Deep lacerations to the foot or hand, crush injuries, a mechanism in which foreign bodies may be buried in the tissue, and penetrating wounds of unknown depth should be referred as well. Other considerations include whether the injury location dictates the need for added repairing skill owing to concerns of postrepair cosmesis, or if the physician is simply uncomfortable with the potential repair. In these cases, the patient should be referred to the emergency department.[23]

## Suturing

- Wound irrigation has classically been done with sterile saline, yet a recent Cochrane review indicated that tap water does not increase the risk of infection.[24] Copiously rinse the wound with the aim to clean and dilute bacterial load. This can be done by placing the wound under a running faucet or with a 30 mL syringe and a 19-gauge needle.[23]
- It is considered safe to use clean, nonsterile examination gloves as opposed to sterile gloves during wound repair because it has been shown to have little to no effect of the rate of infection.[25]
- Anesthetize the area using local injectable agents such as such as 1% to 2% lidocaine or 0.25% bupivacaine. Anesthetics with epinephrine can be considered to help with bleeding and seem to be safe in digits and extremities at appropriate dilutions.[22]
- The exact suture method varies according to the location, size, and shape of the laceration. Helpful tips to keep in mind include[23]:
  - Nonabsorbable nylon monofilament (Ethilon) sutures are typically used to close superficial layers of skin.
  - For deeper lacerations, simply closing the superficial layers is inadequate because this procedure can create potential spaces at risk of infection or creation of excessive tension across the laceration. To reapproximate these deeper layers, use absorbable sutures such as polyglactin 910 (Vicryl) and poliglecaprone 25 (Monocryl).
  - The suture needle should penetrate the skin perpendicular to the wound edge, and at 90° to the skin surface (**Fig. 8**).
  - A suturing technique using a smooth twist of the wrist will evert the edges of the laceration on closure. Upon healing, this technique minimizes the effect of scar retraction and improves cosmesis.

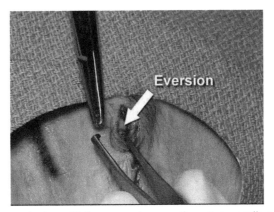

**Fig. 8.** Evert the wound edge with forceps and ensure the suture needle enters the skin in a perpendicular fashion. (*From* Thomsen TW, Lammers RL. Laceration Repair: Simple Interrupted Sutures. (Procedures Consult/ Clinical Key/ Last updated: 5/14/17).; with permission.)

- For cosmetic reasons, an effort should be made to use the finest suture possible (**Table 3**)
- The application of an antibiotic ointment including neomycin or bacitracin after suture closure has been shown to decrease the rate of infection.[22]

### Adhesive

Not all lacerations require suturing for adequate healing and, in certain cases, an adhesive or adhesive strips may be used. A Cochrane review revealed that adhesives yield similar outcomes to suturing when comparing procedure time, pain, complications, and cosmesis.[26] The 2 varieties most available are *n*-butyl-1-cyanoacrylate (Histoacryl Blue, PeriAcryl) and 2-octyl cyanoacrylate (Dermabond, Surgiseal).[22] Indications for use include clean, simple, and shallow linear lacerations that are well-approximated and not under tension. Adhesive strips, applied perpendicularly to the wound to obtain closure, are an excellent alternative and have been determined to be the most cost-effective closure technique for low-tension wounds.[27]

Regardless of the method of wound approximation, the area should be covered with a clean dry gauze and kept covered for at least 12 to 24 hours. Cover the region with an occlusive or semiocclusive dressing or gauze with petroleum gel for wounds with drainage. Replace every 48 hours or if saturated. Sutures should be removed according to their location (**Box 2**). In clean and simple lacerations, there is no need for systemic antibiotics; however, this recommendation changes if the wound is complex, deep, involving a joint, or involves a bite or puncture wound. Furthermore, in patients sustaining these higher risk injuries, it is important to review the tetanus vaccination status. A tetanus booster is indicated if more than 5 years has elapsed since the previous booster. However, if the vaccination status is uncertain or the individual never completed the entire 3-dose vaccine series, then a tetanus immunoglobulin is warranted.

### Nail Removal

A procedure regularly completed in the medical training room is a partial or complete nail excision. The most common indication for this procedure is an ingrown toenail or onychocryptosis. This painful condition can result from the improper trimming of nails, trauma, unsuitable footwear, hyperhidrosis, or increased mechanical or external

**Table 3**
**Suture size and timing of removal**

| Body Part | Suture Size | Timing of Removal |
|-----------|-------------|-------------------|
| Trunk<br>Feet | 3-0 | 8–10 d[a] |
| Limbs<br>Scalp<br>Scalp | 4-0 | 7–8 d[a] |
| Face<br>Hand | 5-0 | 3–5 d[a] then apply skin tape |
| Ear<br>Lip<br>Eyelid | 6-0, 7-0 | 3–5 d then apply skin tape |

[a] Add 2 to 4 d to the timing of removal if laceration is across a mobile joint.

*Adapted from* Forsch RT. Laceration repair (procedure). [Updated 2018 Nov19]. Essential Evidence Plus. http://www.essentialevidenceplus.com/content/eee/615. Accessed December 17, 2018; with permission.

pressures to the foot.[28] Additional indications for nail removal include unsuccessful attempts at treating onychomycosis both topically and orally, as well as recurrent paronychia. Initially, attempts at conservative management including warm water soaks, cotton wick insertion to the nail edges, and gentle soft tissue retraction are recommended. However, if there is continued dysfunction or pain, partial or full removal of the nail is recommended.

### Evaluation

There exists a range of severities with onychocryptosis. More mild cases will have some soft tissue edema, pain, and erythema along the lateral nail edge adjacent

**Box 2**
**Criteria for use of tissue adhesives**

Wound less than 12 hours old

Linear (not stellate)

Hemostatic

Not crossing a joint

Not crossing a mucocutaneous junction

Not in a hair-bearing area (unless hair apposition technique is being used)

Not under significant tension (or tension relieved with deep absorbable sutures)

Not grossly contaminated

Not infected

Not devitalized

Not a result of mammalian bite

No chronic condition that might impair wound healing

*Reprinted* with permission from Laceration Repair: A Practical Approach, May 15, 2017, Vol 95, No 10, American Family Physician. Copyright © 2017 American Academy of Family Physicians. All Rights Reserved.

to the affected nail. Symptoms can progress into increased edema, seropurulent drainage and infection. If left untreated, a more permanent nail-fold hypertrophy with adjacent granulation tissue may be noted.[29] For partial nail resection[30] (**Fig. 9**):

- Position patient such that the hand/foot is resting completely on the table.
- Cleanse the affected digit with iodine and alcohol.
- Complete a digit nerve block using 6 to 8 mL of lidocaine or bupivacaine. Formulations without epinephrine are traditionally used, yet evidence exists supporting the safety of anesthetics containing epinephrine in digits at the proper dilution.[22] Smaller gauge needles (25 gauge, 27 gauge) are recommended.
- (Optional): Consider a tourniquet or rubber band for hemostasis. Apply for the shortest period possible.
- Gently insert a nail elevator underneath the lateral edge (~25%) of the nail to be removed, ensuring the nail completely separates from the nail bed. It is important to extend this underneath the nail fold to release the lateral horns of the nail.
- Use bandage scissors to cut the nail from the distal, free edge proximally toward the cuticle and under the nail fold. One will feel a release when completely through the nail plate.
- Using a hemostat or clamp, grip the avulsed nail fragment to grasp as much of the nail as possible in the instrument. Retract in a steady and outward motion toward the lateral nail taking care to remove the entire fragment. If the nail plate breaks, grasp the remaining nail and reattempt.
- Release the tourniquet.
- Consider destruction of the nail-forming matrix:
  - Phenolization: Administer a solution of 80% to 88% phenol to the affected nail matrix for 30 seconds, taking care to avoid the remaining nail bed or surrounding tissues. Repeat this process twice more. Irrigate the area well with 70% isopropyl alcohol to neutralize the phenol.
    - Nail removal coupled with the application of phenol decreases the risk of recurrence when compared with a simple nail removal alone.[31]
    - The use of phenol increases the risk of postintervention infection.[32]
    - Direct surgical excision or use of electrocautery, carbon dioxide laser, or radiofrequency ablation can be considered to remove any granulation tissue present. These methods have been shown to be equally or less effective than phenol application regarding recurrence and infection.[30]

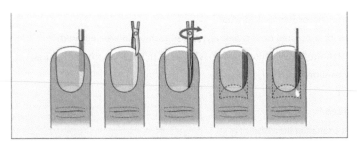

**Fig. 9.** Partial nail resection. An elevator is used to elevate and free the affected side of the nail, before cutting it with a splitter or scissors. Grasp the avulsed piece and rotate while retracting. Ensure the entire nail is removed. Consider phenolizing or chemical cauterization. (*From* Richert, B; Rich, P. Nail Surgery. In Bolognia JL et al. Dermatology, 4th Ed., 2017. Elsevier; with permission.)

- Apply antibacterial ointment (ie, bacitracin/polymyxin), cover with a sterile gauze, and secure with a bandage. Daily cleansing with repeat application of new bandaging is recommended.
- Avoid strenuous physical activity for 1 week.
- Monitor for infection. Antibiotics are not indicated prophylactically in most cases because removal of the irritant nail is sufficient.

### Complete nail removal

Follow the steps for the partial nail removal with a few modifications:

- Elevate the entire nail plate from the nail bed.
- Grasp firmly and retract steadily while securing the digit and moving the nail in a lateral then medial motion in attempts to remove the entire nail fold corners.
- Alternatively, one may cut down the middle of the nail plate and remove the nail in 2 steps, each retracting toward the nail's lateral edge.

## Nail Trephination

A second nail condition not uncommon to sports medicine is a subungual hematoma. The highly vascular nature of a nail bed proves to be a particularly susceptible area to bleeding with either blunt or sharp trauma. Bleeding gets trapped under a nail plate resulting in the formation of a hematoma, which creates pressure and significant discomfort. Decompression of the hematoma by trephination—the creation of a small hole in the nail—provides a path for the blood to evacuate. This procedure relieves the pressure and thus the pain.

### Evaluation

Again, it is imperative to take a thorough history and physical. Caution should be taken to ensure a cause and effect relationship to the hematoma.[33,34] If such a relationship cannot be identified, the nail finding may represent a different condition, including melanoma, Kaposi's sarcoma, junctional nevus, or other dermatologic findings. If a traumatic etiology is identified, it may indicate a fracture of the underlying distal phalanx; a comorbid condition is present in 50% of these injuries.[35] A fracture must not be discounted because, theoretically, trephination of a nail converts a closed tuft fracture to an open fracture. A bluish-black discoloration underneath a nail is seen on physical examination, with exacerbation of pain on palpation. Attention should be placed on quantifying the percentage of the nail affected by the hematoma, as well as any injury to the nail margins. If the nail is split or a nail bed laceration exists, the patient should be referred to a specialist for repair. Document sensation and capillary refill to the digit as well as the functionality of the flexor and extensor tendons. Any concern beyond that of a simple subungual hematoma warrants referral to a hand surgeon for further examination and consideration of radiographic evaluation.

To trephinate a subungual hematoma (**Fig. 10**):

- Clean the nail and finger thoroughly and place onto a sterile field.
- Ensure universal precautions are followed (a sudden release of pressure on the hematoma can result in a spray of blood).
- Apply a portable hot cautery to the center of the hematoma. Activate the heat in short 3- to 4-second increments while applying gentle pressure to the nail. Feel for the release as the cautery completes the nail transection. Immediately stop any pressure so as not to damage the nail bed.

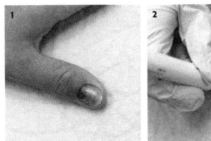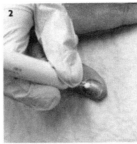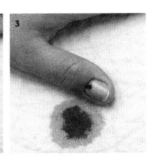

**Fig. 10.** Nail trephination. (1) Position the digit to support the nail, and cleanse. (2) Apply gentle pressure with cautery device in small time increments until a "give" is appreciated. (3) The drained hematoma will result in pain relief. (*From* Ambrose G, Berlin D. Incision and Drainage (Ch 37). In: Roberts and Hedges' Clinical Procedures in Emergency Medicine and Acute Care, Elsevier; 738-773.e4; with permission.)

- Gently apply pressure to the surrounding soft tissues to evacuate the blood. The nail will resume a more normal, pink color.
- Clean and dry the nail before applying a sterile dry dressing. Keep the digit dry for 48 hours.

Other methods to trephinate include using an unwound paperclip sterilized with a flame or using a sterile needle. These techniques yield smaller holes so will likely require more than one for successful evacuation and to minimize chances that the hematoma will reaccumulate.

### Auricular Hematoma Evacuation

Ear trauma is a common finding across sports, particularly those with contact such as wrestling, boxing, rugby, and mixed martial arts.[36] The most frequently encountered injury to the ear is the formation of an auricular hematoma otherwise referred to as a cauliflower ear or wrestler's ear. Although there have been no good quality trials completed regarding management techniques, it is generally agreed that prompt evacuation of the hematoma with attempts to prevent reaccumulation is preferred over leaving it untreated.[36,37]

The outer ear, or the auricle, protrudes from the head leaving it in a susceptible location to trauma. It is composed of a delicate layer of perichondrium overlying a thin layer of cartilage. This perichondrium provides perfusion to the cartilage, supplying essential nutrients. Blunt trauma to this region can produce shearing forces resulting in the formation of a hematoma located between the perichondrial skin layer and this cartilage. A disruption of these 2 layers affects both the healing potential as well as the appearance of the ear (**Fig. 11**). It is important to address these hematomas promptly to preserve as much of the cartilage as possible, preferably within 6 hours of the trauma.[36] Alternatively, if a hematoma is left unattended, this can result in infection, cartilage necrosis, and a disfiguring fibrotic deformity resembling the appearance of a cauliflower, thus the term cauliflower ear.

Clinically, an acute auricular hematoma presents as a soft, fluctuant mass and can be located anywhere along the auricle. If located in the concha, this can result in blockage of the ear canal and result in diminished hearing acuity. There is commonly an ecchymotic discoloration and tenderness associated with the skin around the

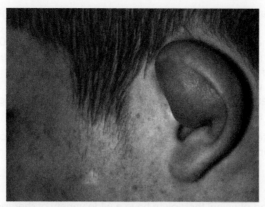

**Fig. 11.** An auricular hematoma, which can block the auditory canal affecting hearing. (*From* Mueller, RV. Facial trauma: Soft tissue injuries (Ch 2). In: Plastic Surgery: Volume 3: Craniofacial, Head and Neck Surgery and Pediatric Plastic Surgery, 2, Elsevier; 22-46.e4; with permission.)

perimeter. The more time that passes after the trauma, the more likely the hematoma will begin to clot, resulting in a firmer collection. Once days to weeks have passed, this becomes the firm deformity that comprises a classic cauliflower ear.

### *Evaluation*

It is imperative to complete a thorough examination of the head and neck, because any trauma that can result in a hematoma can also result in a less obvious head injury, internal ear disruption (ie, tympanic membrane rupture), or a concussion. To decompress small, acute hematomas:

- Cleanse area with antiseptic such as betadine and alcohol.
- Apply anesthesia such as lidocaine 1% if desired by the patient using a small needle (25 gauge, 27 gauge). Often, this step is not necessary because adding more fluid to an already taut swelling will result in more discomfort. Nonpharmacologic methods such as cognitive distraction have been found to be effective.
- Gently introduce an 18-gauge needle into the most fluctuant, dependent area of the hematoma at an acute angle to the ear, ensuring there is no further penetration of the cartilage.
- Aspirate while milking the hematoma to ensure maximal drainage.
- Remove the needle and immediately apply pressure for 10 minutes followed by the application of pressure dressing.

For large, subacute hematomas, consider incision and drainage.[36,38]

- Cleanse the area with an antiseptic such as betadine and alcohol.
- Apply local anesthesia with lidocaine 1% without epinephrine.
- Incise the hematoma in line with the curve of the auricle at the most dependent part of the hematoma using an 11 blade. For cosmetic purposes, attempt to maintain the incision parallel to the helical curve.[38]
- Using sterile hemostats, gently and bluntly gain access into the hematoma pocket and remove the clot, taking care to minimize further damage to the perichondrium.
- Irrigate the evacuated pocket with sterile saline.

- Reapproximate the perichondrium and the auricular cartilage. This may be done by:
  - Suturing the incision closed with a mattress stitch using a 5-0 suture (absorbable or nonabsorbable) through the cartilage ensuring the presence of a small window for drainage.
  - Bolstering using a material such as sterile petrolatum gauze or thermoplastic splint material molded to the ear and sutured to the ear using nonabsorbable 3-0 or 4-0 sutures. Bolsters may be removed after a week.

It should be noted that an auricular hematoma is a potentially avoidable condition with the use of appropriate protection and headgear.

## SUMMARY

Athletic trainers and physical therapists have a wide variety of therapeutic modalities, manual therapy techniques, and rehabilitation exercises at their disposal. To choose the most effective treatment for each specific athletic condition and stage of recovery, it is important to have an understanding of the scientific rationale for each modality. Similarly, because it is impossible to predict the cases a sports medicine physician will encounter in the athletic training room or on the sidelines, a familiarity with the management of common conditions and the use of procedures, as appropriate, is essential to the provision of high-level care regardless of the clinical situation.

## REFERENCES

1. Malanga GA, Yan N, Stark J. Mechanisms and efficacy or heat and cold therapies for musculoskeletal injury. Postgrad Med 2015;127(1):57–65.
2. Logan CA, Asnis PD, Provencher MT. The role of therapeutic modalities in surgical and nonsurgical management of orthopaedic injuries. J Am Acad Orthop Surg 2017 Aug;25(8):556–68.
3. Dupuy O, Douzi W, Theurot D, et al. An evidence-based approach for choosing post-exercise recovery techniques to reduce markers of muscle damage, soreness, fatigue, and inflammation: a systematic review with meta-analysis. Front Physiol 2018;9:403.
4. Hohenauer E, Taeymans J, Baeyens JP, et al. The effect of post-exercise cryotherapy on recovery characteristics: a systematic review and meta-analysis. PLoS One 2015;10(9). https://doi.org/10.1371/journal.pone.0139028.
5. Denegar CR, Saliba E, Saliba S. Therapeutic modalities for musculoskeletal injuries. 2nd edition. Champaign (IL): Human Kinetics; 2006.
6. Bieuzen F, Bleakley CM, Costello JT. Contrast water therapy and exercise induced muscle damage: a systematic review and meta-analysis. PLoS One 2013;8(4):e62356.
7. Desmeules F, Boudreault J, Roy JS, et al. The efficacy of therapeutic ultrasound for rotator cuff tendinopathy: a systematic review and meta-analysis. Phys Ther Sport 2015;16:276–84.
8. Shanks P, Curran M, Fletcher P, et al. The effectiveness of therapeutic ultrasound for musculoskeletal conditions of the lower limb: a literature review. Foot (Edinb) 2010;20:133–9.
9. Tsai WC, Tang SFT, Liang FC. Effect of therapeutic ultrasound on tendons. Am J Phys Med Rehabil 2011;90:1068–73.

10. Martinez de Albornoz P, Khanna A, Longo UG, et al. The evidence of low-intensity pulsed ultrasound for *in vitro*, animal and human fracture healing. Br Med Bull 2011;100:39–57.

11. Schandelmaier S, Kaushal A, Lytvyn L, et al. Low intensity pulsed ultrasound for bone healing: systematic review of randomized controlled trials. BMJ 2017;356: j656.

12. Haun CT, Roberts MD, Romero MA, et al. Concomitant external pneumatic compression treatment with consecutive days of high intensity interval training reduces markers of proteolysis. Eur J Appl Physiol 2017;117(12):2587–600.

13. Winke M, Williamson S. Comparison of pneumatic compression device to a compression garment during recovery from DOMS. Int J Exerc Sci 2018;11(3): 375–83.

14. Hill J, Howatson G, van Someren K, et al. Compression garments and recovery from exercise-induced muscle damage: a meta-analysis. Br J Sports Med 2014;48:1340–6.

15. Brown F, Gissane C, Howatson G, et al. Compression garments and recovery from exercise: a meta-analysis. Sports Med 2017;47(11):2245–67.

16. Brummitt J. The role of massage in sports performance and rehabilitation: current evidence and future direction. North Am J Sports Phys Ther 2008;3(1):7–21.

17. Weerapong P, Hume P, Kolt G. The mechanisms of massage and effects on performance, muscle recovery, and injury prevention. Sports Med 2005;35(3): 235–56.

18. Cheatham SW, Lee M, Cain M, et al. The efficacy of instrument assisted soft tissue mobilization: a systematic review. J Can Chiropr Assoc 2016;60(3):200–11.

19. Lowe D. Cupping therapy: an analysis of the effects of suction on skin and the possible influence on human health. Complement Ther Clin Pract 2017;29:162–8.

20. Al-Bedah AMN, Elsubai IS, Qureshi NA, et al. The medical perspective of cupping therapy: effects and mechanisms of action. J Tradit Complement Med 2018;1–8. https://doi.org/10.1016/j.jtcme.2018.03.003.

21. Dunning J, Butts R, Mourad F, et al. Dry needling: a literature review with implications for clinical practice guidelines. Phys Ther Rev 2014;19(4):252–65.

22. Forsch RT, Little SH, Williams C. Laceration repair: a practical approach. Am Fam Physician 2017;95(10):628–36.

23. Forsch RT. Laceration repair (procedure) 2018. Essential Evidence Plus. Available at: http://www.essentialevidenceplus.com/content/eee/615. Accessed December 17, 2018.

24. Fernandez R, Griffiths R. Water for wound cleansing. Cochrane Database Syst Rev 2012;(2):CD003861.

25. Heal C, Sriharan S, Buttner PG, et al. Comparing non-sterile to sterile gloves for minor surgery: a prospective randomised controlled non-inferiority trial. Med J Aust 2015;202(1):27–31.

26. Farion K, Osmond MH, Hartling L, et al. Tissue adhesives for traumatic lacerations in children and adults. Cochrane Database Syst Rev 2002;(3):CD003326.

27. Zempsky WT, Zehrer CL, Lyle CT, et al. Economic comparison of methods of wound closure: wound closure strips vs. sutures and wound adhesives. Int Wound J 2005;2(3):272–81.

28. Zuber TJ. Ingrown toenail removal. Am Fam Physician 2002;65(12):2547–50.

29. Heidelbaugh JJ, Lee H. Management of the ingrown toenail. Am Fam Physician 2009;79(4):303–8.

30. Ebell MH, Lee H, Heidelbaugh J. Toenail removal (procedure). 2017. Essential Evidence Plus. Available at: http://www.essentialevidenceplus.com/content/eee/617. Accessed November 21, 2018.
31. Eekhof JA, Van Wijk B, Knuistingh Neven A, et al. Interventions for ingrowing toenails. Cochrane Database Syst Rev 2012;(4):CD001541.
32. Gerritsma-Bleeker C, Klaase J, Geelkerken R, et al. Partial matrix excision or segmental phenolization for ingrowing toenails. Arch Surg 2002;137:320–5.
33. Ambrose G, Berlin D. Incision and drainage. In: Roberts and Hedges' clinical procedures in emergency medicine and acute care. 7th edition. Elsevier; 2019. p. 738–73. Available at: https://www.clinicalkey.com/#!/content/3-s2.0-B9780323354783000373?scrollTo=%23top.
34. Fastle RK, Bothner J. Subungual hematoma. 2018. Up To Date. Available at: https://www.uptodate.com/contents/subungual-hematoma?. Accessed November 1, 2018.
35. Roser SE, Gellman H. Comparison of nail bed repair versus nail trephination for subungual hematomas in children. J Hand Surg Am 1999;(24):1166–70.
36. Skidmore K, Hatcher JD. Cauliflower ear. In: StatPearls. Treasure Island (FL): StatPearls Publishing; 2018. Available at: https://www.ncbi.nlm.nih.gov/books/NBK470424/. Accessed September 30, 2018.
37. Interventions for acute auricular haematoma. 2011. Cochrane Database of Syst Rev. Essential Evidence Plus. Available at: http://www.essentialevidenceplus.com/content/cochrane/4166#accept. Accessed November 21, 2018.
38. Malloy KM, Hollander JE. Assessment and management of auricular hematoma and cauliflower ear. 2017. Up To Date. Available at: https://www.uptodate.com/contents/assessment-and-management-of-auricular-hematoma-and-cauliflower-ear. Accessed November 21, 2018.

# UNITED STATES POSTAL SERVICE®

## Statement of Ownership, Management, and Circulation
### (All Periodicals Publications Except Requester Publications)

| 1. Publication Title | 2. Publication Number | 3. Filing Date |
|---|---|---|
| CLINICS IN SPORTS MEDICINE | 000 – 702 | 9/18/2019 |

| 4. Issue Frequency | 5. Number of Issues Published Annually | 6. Annual Subscription Price |
|---|---|---|
| JAN, APR, JUL, OCT | 4 | $364.00 |

7. Complete Mailing Address of Known Office of Publication (Not printer) (Street, city, county, state, and ZIP+4®)

ELSEVIER INC.
230 Park Avenue, Suite 800
New York, NY 10169

Contact Person
STEPHEN R. BUSHING

Telephone (Include area code)
215-239-3688

8. Complete Mailing Address of Headquarters or General Business Office of Publisher (Not printer)

ELSEVIER INC.
230 Park Avenue, Suite 800
New York, NY 10169

9. Full Names and Complete Mailing Addresses of Publisher, Editor, and Managing Editor (Do not leave blank)

Publisher (Name and complete mailing address)

TAYLOR BALL, ELSEVIER INC.
1600 JOHN F KENNEDY BLVD. SUITE 1800
PHILADELPHIA, PA 19103-2899

Editor (Name and complete mailing address)

LAUREN BOYLE, ELSEVIER INC.
1600 JOHN F KENNEDY BLVD. SUITE 1800
PHILADELPHIA, PA 19103-2899

Managing Editor (Name and complete mailing address)

PATRICK MANLEY, ELSEVIER INC.
1600 JOHN F KENNEDY BLVD. SUITE 1800
PHILADELPHIA, PA 19103-2899

10. Owner (Do not leave blank. If the publication is owned by a corporation, give the name and address of the corporation immediately followed by the names and addresses of all stockholders owning or holding 1 percent or more of the total amount of stock. If not owned by a corporation, give the names and addresses of the individual owners. If owned by a partnership or other unincorporated firm, give its name and address as well as those of each individual owner. If the publication is published by a nonprofit organization, give its name and address.)

| Full Name | Complete Mailing Address |
|---|---|
| WHOLLY OWNED SUBSIDIARY OF REED/ELSEVIER, US HOLDINGS | 1600 JOHN F KENNEDY BLVD. SUITE 1800 PHILADELPHIA, PA 19103-2899 |

11. Known Bondholders, Mortgagees, and Other Security Holders Owning or Holding 1 Percent or More of Total Amount of Bonds, Mortgages, or Other Securities. If none, check box. → ☐ None

| Full Name | Complete Mailing Address |
|---|---|
| N/A | |

12. Tax Status (For completion by nonprofit organizations authorized to mail at nonprofit rates) (Check one)
The purpose, function, and nonprofit status of this organization and the exempt status for federal income tax purposes:
☒ Has Not Changed During Preceding 12 Months
☐ Has Changed During Preceding 12 Months (Publisher must submit explanation of change with this statement)

PS Form **3526**, July 2014 [Page 1 of 4 (see instructions page 4)] PSN 7530-01-000-9931    PRIVACY NOTICE: See our privacy policy on www.usps.com.

---

| 13. Publication Title | | 14. Issue Date for Circulation Data Below |
|---|---|---|
| CLINICS IN SPORTS MEDICINE | | JULY 2019 |

| 15. Extent and Nature of Circulation | | | Average No. Copies Each Issue During Preceding 12 Months | No. Copies of Single Issue Published Nearest to Filing Date |
|---|---|---|---|---|
| a. Total Number of Copies (Net press run) | | | 181 | 190 |
| b. Paid Circulation (By Mail and Outside the Mail) | (1) | Mailed Outside-County Paid Subscriptions Stated on PS Form 3541 (Include paid distribution above nominal rate, advertiser's proof copies, and exchange copies) | 102 | 117 |
| | (2) | Mailed In-County Paid Subscriptions Stated on PS Form 3541 (Include paid distribution above nominal rate, advertiser's proof copies, and exchange copies) | 0 | 0 |
| | (3) | Paid Distribution Outside the Mails Including Sales Through Dealers and Carriers, Street Vendors, Counter Sales, and Other Paid Distribution Outside USPS® | 27 | 38 |
| | (4) | Paid Distribution by Other Classes of Mail Through the USPS (e.g., First-Class Mail®) | 0 | 0 |
| c. Total Paid Distribution (Sum of 15b (1), (2), (3), and (4)) | | ► | 129 | 155 |
| d. Free or Nominal Rate Distribution (By Mail and Outside the Mail) | (1) | Free or Nominal Rate Outside-County Copies included on PS Form 3541 | 41 | 22 |
| | (2) | Free or Nominal Rate In-County Copies Included on PS Form 3541 | 0 | 0 |
| | (3) | Free or Nominal Rate Copies Mailed at Other Classes Through the USPS (e.g., First-Class Mail) | 0 | 0 |
| | (4) | Free or Nominal Rate Distribution Outside the Mail (Carriers or other means) | 0 | 0 |
| e. Total Free or Nominal Rate Distribution (Sum of 15d (1), (2), (3) and (4)) | | ► | 41 | 22 |
| f. Total Distribution (Sum of 15c and 15e) | | ► | 170 | 177 |
| g. Copies not Distributed (See Instructions to Publishers #4 (page #3)) | | ► | 11 | 13 |
| h. Total (Sum of 15f and g) | | ► | 181 | 190 |
| i. Percent Paid (15c divided by 15f times 100) | | ► | 75.88% | 87.57% |

* If you are claiming electronic copies, go to line 16 on page 3. If you are not claiming electronic copies, skip to line 17 on page 3.

| 16. Electronic Copy Circulation | | Average No. Copies Each Issue During Preceding 12 Months | No. Copies of Single Issue Published Nearest to Filing Date |
|---|---|---|---|
| a. Paid Electronic Copies | ► | | |
| b. Total Paid Print Copies (Line 15c) + Paid Electronic Copies (Line 16a) | ► | | |
| c. Total Print Distribution (Line 15f) + Paid Electronic Copies (Line 16a) | ► | | |
| d. Percent Paid (Both Print & Electronic Copies) (16b divided by 16c × 100) | ► | | |

☒ I certify that 50% of all my distributed copies (electronic and print) are paid above a nominal price.

17. Publication of Statement of Ownership

☒ If the publication is a general publication, publication of this statement is required. Will be printed ☐ Publication not required.
in the  OCTOBER 2019  issue of this publication.

18. Signature and Title of Editor, Publisher, Business Manager, or Owner

*Stephen R. Bushing*    Date  9/18/2019

STEPHEN R. BUSHING - INVENTORY DISTRIBUTION CONTROL MANAGER

I certify that all information furnished on this form is true and complete. I understand that anyone who furnishes false or misleading information on this form or who omits material or information requested on the form may be subject to criminal sanctions (including fines and imprisonment) and/or civil sanctions (including civil penalties).

PS Form **3526**, July 2014 (Page 3 of 4)    PRIVACY NOTICE: See our privacy policy on www.usps.com

# Moving?

## Make sure your subscription moves with you!

To notify us of your new address, find your **Clinics Account Number** (located on your mailing label above your name), and contact customer service at:

Email: journalscustomerservice-usa@elsevier.com

800-654-2452 (subscribers in the U.S. & Canada)
314-447-8871 (subscribers outside of the U.S. & Canada)

Fax number: 314-447-8029

Elsevier Health Sciences Division
Subscription Customer Service
3251 Riverport Lane
Maryland Heights, MO 63043

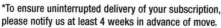

*To ensure uninterrupted delivery of your subscription, please notify us at least 4 weeks in advance of move.

ELSEVIER

Printed and bound by CPI Group (UK) Ltd, Croydon, CR0 4YY

08/05/2025

01864743-0001